Body, Mind and the B Vitamins

by Ruth Adams

and

Frank Murray

Larchmont Books

NEW YORK

Fifth Printing: November, 1977
Fourth Printing: November 1976
Third Printing: June 1975
Second Printing: June 1973
First Printing: June 1972

Contents

Foreword

TWENTY YEARS AGO only the most foolhardy psychiatrists would have considered that nutrition, except possibly for starvation, played any significant roles in the etiology and treatment of mental diseases. These concepts were novel to the field of general medicine, and, even today, there are very few medical colleges where adequate courses on nutrition and its clinical applications are taught. Dr. Jean Mayer has recently stated that the average physician knows about as much as his secretary, and that if she is overweight she probably knows somewhat more.

In the field of psychiatry, psychoanalysis had just completed its take-over of the American Psychiatric Association, it was beginning to complete its sweep of University Departments of Psychiatry, which succumbed a little later, and it had initiated take-over of the editorships of the psychiatric journals. Psychoanalysis had absolutely no use for the field of nutrition, nor did it even consider that patients had a body. In fact, about twenty years ago Dr. Manfred Bleuler, son of the famous Eugene Bleuler, forecast that in the foreseeable future no further biochemical research into the etiology of schizophrenia would be done. I am certain that he would have made the same statement about nutritional research playing any useful role in psychiatry.

However, today the situation is different. Psychiatrists no longer deny the biochemical basis of schizophrenia, even if they only pay lip service to this idea. The recent formation of the Academy of Orthomolecular Psychiatry, which held its first annual scientific meeting in Dallas, Texas in 1972, foreshadows what will be the future role of nutrition in the general field of psychiatry and, hopefully, in medicine. It is clear that at last the total environment, not only the psychosocial but also the nutritional environment, is beginning to be examined in its proper context.

This change in opinion closely parallels my own personal experience with psychiatry. I had started out as a Ph.D. in biochemistry, but, in my first year of psychiatry, I was very interested in psychoanalytic theory. My treatment at that time was directed toward psychodynamic psychotherapy, including individual psychotherapy, psychodrama and group psychotherapy. For the next ten years of my life as a psychiatrist, my orientation swung over very markedly toward a broad genetic biochemical point of view, but only in the past ten years have I begun to give proper consideration to the vast importance of nutritional factors.

At present it is my conclusion that if every general practitioner who refers patients to me were to practice the principles of orthomolecular psychiatry; that is, the proper incorporation of nutritional theory and practice into psychiatric treatment, I would immediately lose 85% of my practice. It sometimes appears to me that I am no longer practicing psychiatry as it is practiced by the majority of psychiatrists, but have become an internist specializing in nutritional medicine with a special skill in psychiatry.

It is interesting to speculate on the factors which have led to this great transformation which has affected a small number of psychiatrists and which will undoubtedly affect the majority over the next two decades. Biochemical nutritionists were very helpful, *e.g.* Adelle Davis and Dr. Carlton Fredericks, who have done a good deal to popularize the importance of adequate nutrition to the public. Dr. John Yudkin has done a good deal of work relating the pathological effect of modern diet to its sucrose content. There is no doubt that a good deal of malnutrition is produced by the excessive consumption of sucrose, which not only imbalances the ratio between carbohydrates, protein and fats, but also deprives the patient of essential vitamins and minerals. It does not carry within itself its proper quota of these essential nutrients.

Professor Roger J. Williams, discoverer of pantothenic acid and other vitamins, has pioneered the concept that individuals are biochemically different and that this must be taken into account in the treatment of patients. He has pointed out that chemicals which are ingested into the body become part of the internal environment of the cells. Each person has his own optimum internal environment and he must be aware of what this is wherever possible, and apply the proper nutritional knowledge to maintain optimum stability.

Professor Linus Pauling has provided a theoretic basis for the main principles of orthomolecular psychiatry and has allowed biochemists to understand why some individuals might require huge quantities of certain nutrients; for example, vitamins, in comparison to other individuals. Dr. Irwin Stone has provided an excellent summary of the literature on ascorbic acid, and has pointed to the enormous importance in using adequate quantities. His concept of hypoascorbemia; that is, a genetic disease which afflicts every person alive, is an extremely important one.

Several physicians have also been in the forefront in bringing the importance of nutrition to the attention of society. The first is Dr. William Kaufman, who first pointed out the importance of vitamin B3 in the treatment of various forms of arthritis. Unfortunately, his work has not been duplicated in a controlled sense, although a large number of physicians have used his treatment with great success. Secondly Dr. Fred R. Klenner, who has done an amazing amount of work in proving the importance of huge quantities of ascorbic acid, and, of course, Dr. Evan Shute, who has done similar work in connection with alphatocopherol, a vitamin E component which may be essential in preventing cardiovascular diseases. Finally, we have to take cognizance of Dr. Carl Reich, who has been working with megadoses of vitamin A and D in combination with calcium for the treatment of asthma and has been achieving a good deal of success with this treatment.

Psychiatrists who have been active in this field are Dr. Jonathon Gould, who demonstrated the importance of large quantities of the B vitamins, plus ascorbic acid, in the treatment of certain organic psychoses and delirious states, and, of course, the work I have done with Dr. Humphrey Osmond beginning in 1952, when we ran the first controlled double-blind studies to establish the efficacy of vitamin B3; that is, nicotinic acid or nicotinamide in the treatment of schizophrenia.

There have also been new ideas developed which have been very helpful in popularizing nutrition amongst the medical profession. The first is a concept of the balanced diet put forward by Roger Williams. His work suggests that not only is it important to provide an optimum balance within any one day, but also it is important that each meal be balanced so that the nutrients are absorbed at approximately the same time, and, furthermore, that each particular food ought to be as balanced as possible. From this point of view white bread is not as good as whole-wheat bread, even though white bread consumed with other components in the diet might not be quite as bad as white bread consumed all by itself.

The concept that each total food must carry its own complement of vitamins and minerals is an an extremely useful one, and if generally adopted would prevent the continued sale of many of our prepared foods. The concept of ingesting foods at regular intervals in small quantities has been popularized by physicians like Dr. E. M. Abrahamson, who has been particularly concerned with the concept of hyperinsulinism. Certainly it is well known now that patients and people in general ought to eat three small meals a day, at least, with frequent snacks in between, and that even the best balanced meal in itself, provided only one meal a day is consumed, is not conducive to good health.

Another concept which has come into being is that of the vitamin dependency conditions. A vitamin deficiency disease is produced when a particular factor is lacking in the diet; for example, if there is insufficient nicotinic acid in one's diet, the disease pellagra will occur. However, it is now certain, because of the wide individuality of people, that even though 20 milligrams of nicotinic acid might be adequate for one person, it is possible that 100 or even more milligrams per day might be required for another person. A person who requires 100 milligrams a day and receives 50 is still suffering from a relative deficiency of nicotinic acid, even though 50 milligrams a day would be more than adequate for the majority of our population. We are, therefore, dealing with the concept of dependency conditions where the error is in the person's physiology and not particularly in his diet.

It is also clear now that there are two main kinds of dependencies. There is the dependency which is acquired by living with a diet which is deficient for a long period of time, and there is the dependency which is present early in life which is perhaps genetic. Recently I have examined a small number of Canadian soldiers who were held in a Japanese prison-of-war camp for 44 months. During this time they lost one-third of their body weight and developed severe malnutrition with pellagra, beriberi, scurvy and perhaps other vitamin deficiencies.

Upon returning to Canada they were given what was then considered massive dosages of vitamins, but which would today be considered rather small doses. In any event, they did not fully recover, although their weight came back to normal. Since that time they have suffered from an amazing amount and degree of various psychiatric and physical disabilities. However, the few patients who have come under my care, and who have been placed upon orthomolecular doses of nicotinic acid and vitamin C, have recovered and as far as I can tell have been normal as long as they continue to take the large dosages of nicotinic acid. This is an example of an acquired vitamin dependency.

It was well known to the early pellagrologists that chronic pellagrins would never recover on small dosages of vitamin B3, and it was remarked that they required 600 milligrams per day. Whenever the dose went down below this level, the symptoms of pellagra recurred. This is a dose which is still 60 times as great as what the average nutritionist has recommended to prevent pellagra from occurring. The dependency concept followed the use of megadoses of vitamins which was introduced by the men already listed before.

As for new concepts, certain diseases have

been singled out for special attention; for example, schizophrenia with which I am most familiar. Dr. Osmond and I began our first double-blind experiments (controlled) in 1952 and have since then completed at least four double-blind controlled studies. I, myself, have experience on over 2,000 schizophrenic patients that I have treated since that time, and have been treating them at an accelerating pace since going into private practice in the middle of 1967. On the basis of my own experience going back two decades, and upon the experience of my colleagues in the Academy of Orthomolecular Psychiatry, who have now treated many thousands of cases, it is possible to conclude that the Orthomolecular Approach is the most effective treatment approach there is today for the treatment of schizophrenia.

According to Dr. Loren Mosher, Chief of the Section of Schizophrenia for the National Institute of Mental Health in the year 1970, only 23% of all schizophrenics treated in the United States were thereafter able to work in the community. Since this would be the best criteria of recovery, one can say that only 23% of all schizophrenics treated in the United States recovered to the point where they were able to work. This is still a very low recovery rate and does not even match the so called one-third recovery rate which has been quoted for the past 200 years as characteristic of schizophrenia. However, the Orthomolecular Approach has produced 90% recovery rates on patients who have been sick for a year or less, provided the total program is followed, as has been described many times, and for a period of time to make sure that the optimum time for treatment has been used.

So far there isn't a single study where the technique used as described has failed to yield the same kind of data. There have been several superficial studies where minor aspects of the total program were examined and where the authors failed to confirm; however, this is not surprising. The first rule of science is that when an investigator wishes to corroborate another study he in fact does so. Once this essential fact is hammered home to all our investigators in the field of psychiatry, then the question of lack of reproducibility of data will quickly vanish.

The water-soluble vitamins appear to be especially related to psychiatric syndrome, and, for this reason, this book, entitled *Body, Mind, and the B Vitamins,* will be particularly helpful. So far it seems to me that we can draw the following relationship between vitamins and psychiatric symptoms; (1) Thiamine, whose absence would lead to irritability and depression, (2) Riboflavin, whose absence might lead to disorders of muscular movement, (3) Vitamin B3, whose absence would lead to pellagra and schizophrenia, (4) Vitamin B6, whose absence would lead to epilepsy and schizophrenia, and (5) Vitamin B12, whose absence would lead to the well known anemias but might also lead to chronic fatigue states.

It is interesting that every one of these water-soluble vitamins must be converted into a coenzyme. This requires the addition of phosphate groups at one stage or another. It is quite possible that there is an essential difficulty in phosphorylation or that certain enzymes involved are defective. If this were the case, then one main defect could account for a large variety of conditions depending upon which particular vitamin was mostly affected. Thus, if B1 were not phosphorylated, one might see depression; if B3 were the one most affected, one would see perceptual or thought changes or schizophrenia, and so on.

It is clear that the incidence of degenerative diseases which have been related to western civilization has been growing at a rapid rate. It seems pretty clear to anyone who has observed this phenomena that the usual form of medical practice will not adequately deal with it. The average American diet is too heavily loaded with sucrose, too heavily loaded with refined foods and contains insufficient quantities of vitamins and minerals. If we are ever going to bring this huge problem under control, it will have to be done by raising the general level of nutritional knowledge and information. For this reason books like this one are extremely important and serve a very useful function in alerting society to the importance of these factors.

I suggest that, beginning in public school, classes in nutrition should be given to the students and that these should be continued well into high school. These would not merely be a sterile recitation of the vitamins and what they do but would be an integrated, comprehensive course in which the effect of various nutritional malpractices would be related in terms of health and disease. For example, it could easily be demonstrated in any class that students that come without breakfast are the ones who are going to be most sleepy in the morning and whose marks will be inferior, compared to those students who are following the best nutritional practice.

A. HOFFER, M.D., Ph.D.
Saskatoon, Saskatchewan, Canada.
President, The Huxley Institute for
Biosocial Research,
New York, N. Y.
May 18, 1972

CHAPTER 1

Understanding the B Complex of Vitamins

A NEWBORN BABY lay in convulsions, which many drugs and sedatives had failed to relieve. She was given a single injection of a harmless substance. The convulsions stopped at once. Doctors discovered the child needed injections and tablets daily for the next eight years to prevent further trouble. A child with cystic fibrosis was taking a powerful antibiotic to prevent infections. Neuritis of the nerves of the eye developed as a side effect of the drug. She was given some pills and the neuritis disappeared. The life-saving antibiotic could be administered without harm so long as the other medication was maintained.

A 62-year-old woman came to an Alabama hospital with alarming symptoms. She had no appetite, suffered from nausea and vomiting, mental depression, pallor, muscle pains and heart pains. She had tingling sensations in hands and feet and a scaly dermatitis. She suffered from anemia, exhaustion, swollen ankles, extremely high cholesterol levels and a liver disorder. She had been on a highly nourishing diet to restore her health after a lifetime of heavy drinking. What was wrong? An injection of one harmless substance cured all her symptoms within a few days. This story was told in the *American Journal of Clinical Nutrition.*

Seven young women taking oral contraceptives came to a Florida physician suffering from a desperately serious form of anemia. So long as they took The Pill, the anemia grew worse. The physician gave them a harmless substance in a pill. They improved almost at once and could continue taking The Pill in good health so long as they continued to take the doctor's pill as well. What was it? A wonder drug? This story appeared in the *Journal of the American Medical Association.*

A five-month-old baby was vomiting persistently and had an extensive skin rash which was spreading in spite of many medications his physicians gave him. His breathing was abnormal; he appeared to have acidosis. Put on a new diet, he went into shock. The physicians gave him a bit of one harmless substance. The vomiting stopped immediately and within a few days the baby was completely well. *The Lancet* printed this account.

An acute alcoholic suffering from delirium tremens had not worked for three years, had been alcoholic for six years. He was taken to a New York hospital with an accumulation of fluid in his lungs. In the operating room a tube was inserted into his stomach. Into the tube was poured a liquid food. Within 48 hours the man was walking around, needing no further treatment than the prescribed feeding at regular intervals. After three months he had gained 30 pounds, was working steadily. Magic? Magic doesn't get into medical journals and that's where this story was reported.

A brain-injured child had had seizures every day for three years. His doctors had given him tranquilizers in an effort to control the seizures, with no success. He was given some tablets and eleven days later had his first day completely free from seizures. A second child who had suffered from many seizures every day for two years was completely free from them within three days and was a healthy, happy child four years later. The doctor who treated him believes there may be as many as 20 million American children suffering from varying degrees of mental illness who could be helped with this same therapy. A psychiatrist reported this story in *Schizophrenia*, Volume 3, Number 2.

An 80-year-old widow, living alone since her

husband's death, was depressed, hopeless, suicidal. She suffered from insomnia, was underweight, had an enlarged heart and a peculiar rash on those parts of her face and hands that are exposed to sunlight. She came to a British hospital, was given injections for three weeks, went home, completely well and cheerful.

A patient who had suffered for 20 years from inability to work, loss of interest in surroundings, loss of appetite, food allergies, dizziness, fainting spells, headaches, shortness of breath and nervousness was treated with a certain diet, plus some tablets. Within five days his acute symptoms disappeared, and three months later he was free from all symptoms and leading a well-adjusted life. This story was reported in the *American Journal of Psychiatry.*

A 10-year-old girl, once bright and alert, began to complain of abdominal pains and headaches. Her school grades deteriorated, she became cranky and difficult, refused to play the piano which she had always enjoyed. She heard "voices", felt afraid of many harmless things. Peoples' faces seemed peculiar to her. Buildings appeared to be falling on her. Her physician gave her some tablets and within a month she was once again a bright, happy little girl.

These stories are not fiction. The tablets and injections given, in many instances, are members of the B complex of vitamins, completely harmless and beneficent. The diets that accompanied some of the treatments are diets high in protein and the B vitamins. No wonder drugs are involved; no magic spells. All the stories appeared originally in highly reputable medical and scientific journals, which is where we found them when we were doing research for this book.

This book contains many, many more stories of this kind—just as dramatic, just as convincing. In most of these cases, the B vitamins were given in what is called "megadoses"—that is, amounts much larger than one would ordinarily get at meal times or in food supplements. In some cases, it appears that the vitamin or vitamins involved work like drugs. In others, it is apparent that the individual had need for far more of this particular vitamin than the rest of us need.

In every case, the vitamin treatment is harmless, with none of the unpleasant side effects which accompany many drugs. Is it possible for you to use this information to help yourself or members of your family? With caution, yes, so far as the B vitamins are concerned, for they are water soluble, which means that, if you get more than your body can handle, they are easily and quickly excreted and pose little threat of harm.

It is also our hope that this book, in some small way, can convince more doctors to use vitamins, especially the versatile B Complex, to alleviate much needless suffering.

Better still, with full knowledge of the B Complex, you can probably prevent such widespread disorders that we discuss from ever appearing. That is the purpose of this book—to help you to become acquainted with the B vitamins, what their role is in maintaining good health, what foods they are most abundant in, and how you can use them to secure abundant health for yourself and your family.

When we speak of niacin, riboflavin and thiamine—three of the harmless substances referred to above—we are discussing three of the 11 B vitamins. Unfortunately, most of us know very little about this B Complex, a team of vitamins that work together like mountain climbers, each helping the other out when the need arises. This, then, is one of the few books on all of the B vitamins, their sources, their need in human nutrition, and some of the important research work being done with them.

Although it is possible that more B vitamins will eventually be discovered, U. S. scientists now recognize only eleven. They are:

B-1—Thiamine
B-2—Riboflavin
B-3—Niacin
B-6—Pyridoxine

Pantothenic Acid
Biotin
Folic Acid
B-12—Cobalamine
Choline
Inositol
PABA (Para-amino-benzoic acid)

As you see, some of the B vitamins have numbers and some do not. Also, they skip from B3 to B6, then to B12, etc. Biotin was once called vitamin H. Some books list a B15 which, we are told, is being used most effectively abroad to prevent some serious conditions. One early classic book, *Vitamins in Medicine*, by Dr. Franklin Bicknell and Frederick Prescott, also listed vitamin B12a, B12b, B12c, B13 and B14.

The complexity of vitamin research is well demonstrated by the fact that other substances keep turning up in the B Complex of vitamins which one researcher or another in this country and abroad chooses to call a new vitamin. One such is a vitamin B4 which prevents a disease of poultry, B5 which is essential for health in some animals, B8 also called adenylic acid, B14 which seems to be related to vitamin B12. Whether or not any or perhaps all of these may turn out eventually to be bona fide B vitamins remains to be seen. We know, however, that all these exist in the same foods.

Perhaps we should also add that some biochemists do not regard choline, inositol and PABA as vitamins, although they are part of the B Complex.

Vitamins—any vitamin—do not suddenly appear in a laboratory labeled vitamin B1 or B2. The biochemist does not pick up a cup of brewer's yeast, stir it a little and decide that the big pieces of yeast must be vitamin B1 and the little pieces vitamin B2.

Until about 50 years ago, no one knew there were such things as vitamins, although scientists and physicians knew, in general, that there were some substances in certain foods which could prevent certain deficiency diseases. If the substances were destroyed by heat or soaking or some other process, the disease would not be prevented, no matter how much of the depleted food was eaten. This was what the early scientists had to go on, and they made plenty of mistakes.

Dr. Casimir Funk, who died at 83 in Albany, N. Y. in November 1967, discovered vitamins in 1911. He had theorized that chemical substances, which he called vitamines (from the Latin word "vita" for life and "amine" for chemical compounds containing nitrogen) were capable of preventing deficiency diseases such as scurvy, pellagra and rickets, and indeed were essential to the sustenance of healthy life, according to the Dec. 1, 1967 issue of *Time*. The assumption that all vitamins contained nitrogen later proved to be wrong, and the "e" was dropped from "vitamine."

Moving from the Pasteur Institute in Paris to the Lister Institute of Preventive Medicine in London in 1910, Dr. Funk pursued the causes of beriberi, the vitamin B deficiency disease that attacks the nerves, heart and digestive system. Beriberi was particularly prevalent in those days among Eastern peoples whose diet consisted mainly of polished rice.

Funk put test pigeons on a rice diet, the *Time* article continued. "First he fed them polished rice; then natural rice, with all its bran coating. When the pigeons got the coating they thrived; when they did not they suffered from polyneuritis. Obviously, the bran-fed pigeons were getting a nutrient that the others were not. Funk concentrated the nutrient, now known as vitamin B1."

After becoming a U.S. citizen in 1920, Dr. Funk went back to Europe, where he continued his research in Poland and France. He returned to the U.S. at the start of World War II. "Funk continued his cancer research. . . . All the while, he maintained more than a proprietary interest in nutrition, served as a research consultant to the U.S. Vitamin and Pharmaceutical Corporation, and helped to develop artificial vitamins,"

Time said.

Until 1926 scientists generally believed that vitamin B was a single entity. Then several scientists showed that there were at least two kinds, one of which could be destroyed easily by heat, another which was not destroyed by heat. Soon after, scientists in laboratories in many parts of the world began to isolate different parts of these substances, and, of course, called them by whatever name they happened to think of. Vitamin B2 was called riboflavin, except that in Europe they called it lactoflavine (because it is abundant in milk), and in the U.S. it was called vitamin G for a long time.

What is now pyridoxine has been labeled Factor Y, Factor I, Factor H, adermin and Factor B6. The term "vitamin B complex" at present refers to all vitamins split off from the original vitamin B and identified chemically or by their biological effects. Bicknell and Prescott define a B vitamin as "an organic substance which acts catalytically in all living cells and which is essential for the nutrition of higher animals." A catalyst is a substance which causes biochemical changes to take place. The U.S. Department of Agriculture Handbook, *Food,* defines vitamins as "one group of substances that in relatively small amounts are essential for life and growth."

By "catalytically," Bicknell and Prescott mean that the B vitamins are involved in many of the incredibly complex workings of the body. And we do mean complex. In the official National Academy of Sciences book, *Recommended Dietary Allowances*, the B vitamin biotin is listed as taking part in about 15 or 20 processes involving many different enzymes. Scientists, you see, are not content with just observing that lack of biotin causes certain body symptoms. They must know, too, exactly what biotin does in the body that prevents these symptoms from occurring. Needless to say, scientists have only begun to untangle the mysteries. It may be hundreds of years before all the complexities are understood, or perhaps they never will be.

What we do know, basically and thoroughly, about the B vitamins is that they are indeed a "complex" which means that they are closely related to one another, that they work together and they occur, generally speaking, in the same groups of food.

Thiamine, as we have learned, is the vitamin which prevents beriberi. It is also essential for proper nerve function. Its deficiency brings neuritis, paralysis, atrophy of muscles, edema or swelling. Symptoms disappear magically when thiamine is given.

Riboflavin can bring about a variety of symptoms when it is absent or deficient: mouth inflammation, sores at the corners of the lips, visual fatigue, a "sandy" feeling of the eyes, inability to endure bright lights. Seborrhea, a scaly skin disease, is also a symptom of riboflavin deficiency.

Niacin is responsible for the health of skin, nerves and digestive tract—a big order for a substance needed only in milligrams. Pellagra is the deficiency disease when niacin is lacking. It produces three conditions: Diarrhea, dermatitis and dementia—and death if it is not treated. Niacin is also known as nicotinic acid. Nicotinamide, the physiologically active form of niacin, is also called niacinamide.

Pyridoxine was recently listed by the National Academy of Sciences as being essential to human life and an official recommended dietary allowance was made. Lack of pyridoxine can also cause seborrhea, convulsions in babies, mouth disorders similar to those caused by lack of other B vitamins and nerve symptoms.

Biotin has no number officially. Nor does our NAS set a daily recommended dose, although biotin is assumed to be essential to man. Symptoms of lack of biotin are: lassitude, lack of appetite, depression, muscle pains, scaling dermatitis, nausea, anemia, high blood levels of cholesterol and changes in heart rhythm.

Choline is officially regarded as a vitamin, although no official recommendation for daily intake has been made. In animals it protects against abnormalities in pregnancy and lactation. Lack of it brings anemia, cardiovascular disease and muscle weakness to various animals.

Pantothenic acid, discovered by Dr. Roger J. Williams of the University of Texas, is also involved in many enzyme activities within the body. Lack of this vitamin produces apathy, depression, instability of heart action, abdominal pains, increased susceptibility to infection, impaired function of the important adrenal glands which bulwark us against stress, and certain nerve disorders involving "pins and needles" feelings and muscle weakness. (Do these sound like symptoms of anybody you know?)

Folic acid is closely related in function to vitamin B12. Lack of it produces a kind of anemia (macrocytic) which can be fatal. Symptoms also include inflammation of the tongue, diarrhea, lack of ability to absorb food. It is listed in *Recommended Dietary Allowances* as folacin.

Vitamin B12 is the substance which prevents pernicious anemia. Lack of it causes progressive involvement of the nerves which eventually reaches the spinal cord. Untreated, it is fatal.

Inositol is a substance which occurs along with the rest of the B vitamins. Says *Food,* "It is required for the growth and proper nutrition of animals, but its role in human nutrition is not known." Hence it is not officially a vitamin. Adelle Davis in her book, *Let's Get Well,* says that, in the absence of enough choline and inositol, lecithin cannot be formed in the body. Lecithin is that important emulsifying substance which keeps cholesterol from forming unwanted deposits on the insides of blood vessels. So, although inositol is not officially listed as a B vitamin, it appears that one day it may be.

Para-amino-benzoic acid is sometimes considered a B vitamin, although it is not recognized officially as such. Miss Davis tells us it was available some time ago only on prescription. She tells marvelous stories about its ability to restore color to white hair and says that anyone wanting healthy hair should take large amounts of folic acid, PABA and pantothenic acid daily, as well as using every day wheat germ, liver, brewers yeast and yogurt.

Food states that the sometimes mentioned vitamins B13, B14 and B15 have not been classified as vitamins and have not been proved to be essential to human health. As you can see, these are substances which occur along with the B vitamins, which one scientist or another has isolated and is studying. If someone can come up with proof that one or another of these is actually essential to human life and can prevent the appearance of certain deficiency symptoms, then this substance will probably (after many years of official inquiry) be designated as a vitamin. And that's the way these things are handled.

As we have said, it is unbelievably complex, as everything in nature is. The one certain lesson we can learn from studying the B complex is the lesson our food technologists have never learned and apparently are incapable of learning. Nature likes things whole. Nothing worthwhile is achieved in nature with fragments. Lifting all of the B complex of vitamins from our wholegrain cereals—when they are milled and processed—then returning only bits of three of the B vitamins synthetically is probably the worst possible thing we could do, for the imbalances thus created are unimaginably complex. Many of the trace minerals are also lost in this refining process.

It may take centuries to discover the amount of harm we have done to human health by thus fragmenting one of man's basic foods—bread. Yet this is done by our giant milling industry when they produce white flour, white rice and all the highly processed breakfast cereals.

All the B vitamins occur together in the same foods, although one food may contain a bit more of one, a bit less of another. These foods are:

Liver and all organ meats
Eggs
Milk, cheese
Meat, fish, poultry
Green, leafy vegetables

Whole grains, nuts, seeds, legumes
Food yeast

You can readily see that a diet consisting of just these foods alone is a complete diet, if you add fruits and other vegetables for their vitamin A and vitamin C content. The foods in which the B complex of vitamins are most abundant are also those foods which contain the most protein, so that a diet consisting of the foods listed above, plus fruits and vegetables rich in vitamins A and C, is the best possible diet to follow.

You can also see that, as soon as you begin to dilute this excellent diet with foods made from white refined flours and refined cereals, you lose B vitamins as well as precious minerals. As you add white sugar and foods made from it, you cut down severely on the vitamin B content of your diet, for all vitamins have been removed from the sugarcane to make white sugar. You also create imbalances because Nature has arranged that the B vitamins are essential for the body to process starches and sugars. Yet B vitamins are lacking in these depleted foods. And still we are told that one-half of all food eaten in the U.S. is made up of white flour, processed cereal food and white sugar.

A recent study sponsored by the Agricultural Research Service of the Department of Agriculture, in cooperation with the American Institute of Baking and the Purdue Research Foundation, shows that most of the B complex and vitamin E are lost when wheat is processed into white flour and then made into bread, cake, pasta, etc.

The milling and bleaching of hard and soft wheat for bread and cake strips away 90% of the vitamin E, the report stated. The loss is about 60% in the milling of durum, a variety of hard wheat, for pastas, but there is a further loss in the final processing into macaroni and similar products. As for pyridoxine, the highest loss for the B Complex, less than 15% of the vitamin B6 was retained in bread, 7% in cake, 10 to 20% in crackers and 25% in macaroni.

Speaking before the Subcommittee on Energy, Natural Resources and the Environment in Washington on August 26, 1970, Dr. Henry A. Schroeder of Dartmouth Medical School said: "Most of the trace elements essential for health are removed from processed foods. Unfortunately, they are not restored to the food. The milling of wheat into refined white flour removes 40% of the chromium, 86% of the manganese, 76% of the iron, 89% of the cobalt, 68% of the copper, 78% of the zinc and 48% of the molybdenum, all trace elements essential for life or health," says Dr. Schroeder, a world renowned expert on trace metals.

The B complex must be kept whole, as it is in whole grains, in whole seeds, nuts, eggs, liver, yeast. And when you are buying a B Complex vitamin supplement, make sure it contains all of the B vitamins, as well as some yeast, liver or other rich sources of B vitamins, so that you will also be getting all the other vitamins that may be there but undiscovered, as yet.

CHAPTER 2

Thiamine

A SURVEY RELEASED by the U. S. Department of Agriculture on February 23, 1968 showed that 20% of all American families were eating what the USDA classified as a "poor" diet. The Department's food experts had interviewed 7,500 families and gathered information on all food either bought or home-produced in the preceding week, plus all snacks and meals they had eaten away from home. They graded the food on the basis of the National Academy of Sciences recommendations for daily requirements of calories, protein, the minerals calcium and iron and vitamins A, thiamine, riboflavin and vitamin C. The USDA called a diet "poor" if it supplied less than two-thirds of one or more of the nutrients. For the purposes of this book, we will only mention the statistics as they relate to thiamine and riboflavin. In the Northeast, 9% of the diets were deficient in thiamine; 8% in the North Central, 7% in the south and 10% in the West. For riboflavin, it was 5% in the Northeast, 6% in the North Central, 7% in the South and 6% in the West.

Another survey, this one made by Dr. Arnold Schaefer when he was with the Public Health Service, showed shocking evidence of widespread malnutrition in the U.S. The survey had been amassed after thorough physical examinations of over 83,000 persons. Because the news of widespread malnutrition become so unpleasant to a number of politicians, Dr. Schaefer was forced to resign his post, after more than 15 years of service, and was forbidden to comment on the 10-state survey. It was through the efforts of Senator Ernest Hollings of South Carolina and others that we have been fed additional information from time to time.

At one point it was noted that 9% of those surveyed were short on thiamine, while 19% were getting too little riboflavin. In another report, 11% of all those examined above the poverty level in one state turned out to be deficient or low in vitamin C. The figures on riboflavin are much worse. Below the poverty level, state after state ranges from 5.3% of those deficient or low in the vitamin, up to 31.6% in South Carolina. Above the poverty level, the figure is 23%. So far as ages go, the largest percent of those deficient and low in vitamin B2 occurred among children below six years of age—48.2% in South Carolina.

Beriberi was believed to have been conquered many many years ago. But the *British Medical Journal* for April 10, 1971 reports on two cases of beriberi which occurred in Blackpool, England. Beriberi, the disease of thiamine deficiency, is still prevalent in areas of the world where white rice is eaten almost exclusively, with little in the way of meat, fish or vegetables, which might contribute enough thiamine to prevent the disease.

According to the *Heinz Handbook of Nutrition,* there may be conditions even in the U.S. where so little thiamine is included in the diet that beriberi may result. Chronic alcoholics substitute drinks for foods that contain thiamine. And other conditions increase one's demands for this essential vitamin: pregnancy, breast-feeding, fevers, hyperthyroidism or diseases which interfere with proper absorption or utilization of food (like diarrhea, colitis, etc.) or disorders of the liver.

What are the typical symptoms? The earliest are vague: lack of initiative, lack of appetite, depression, irritability, poor memory, tendency to tire easily and to be unable to concentrate. Then there are vague abdominal and heart complaints. These are symptoms often associated with our senior citizens, especially those who live alone and prepare their own meals.

As the deficiency grows worse, nerves are affected, chiefly in the legs. The victim suffers from neuritis and from a feeling of "pins and needles" in the toes, along with a burning sensation. Arms and fingers are generally affected next. The heart suffers injury resulting in shortness of breath and irregularities of heartbeat. There may also be accumulations of fluid, causing puffy swelling in ankles. The only remedy is large amounts of thiamine—injected, if there is evidence that it will not be thoroughly absorbed.

The two British beriberi patients were admitted to a psychiatric ward. The first was an 80-year-old widow who had lived alone since the death of her husband. She was depressed, slept poorly, ate little, was hopeless about the future and thought frequently of suicide. She was underweight, had a rash on her face and on parts of hands and arms exposed to sunlight—this is another symptom of beriberi. Her chest X-ray showed an enlarged heart.

The second patient was only 48. He had suffered from stomach ulcers and had part of his stomach removed. Because of his wife's death several years before, he also was depressed and apprehensive. He ate little. He could not sleep without barbiturates. His legs were wasted. His ankles showed swelling with fluid.

Both patients were given thiamine by injection and within three weeks depression and swelling had cleared and they had gained weight. They were well physically and mentally and were discharged from the hospital. One can only hope that they were told how easily and inexpensively the symptoms could be prevented —a diet which includes plenty of the foods in which thiamine is abundant plus food supplements containing plenty of all the B vitamins.

The British physician who treated these patients says that the disease may be commoner in England than is generally supposed. He says that vitamin deficiencies there are usually brought on by other factors—disorders of the digestive tract and the mind, alcoholism, poor choices of food, and, among the elderly, social isolation, which leads to loss of appetite and loss of desire to prepare nourishing food.

He goes on to say, "Thiamine deficiency is frequently misdiagnosed and it is noteworthy that the first patient was initially treated for congestive heart failure. Beriberi would probably be frequently recognized if the possibility were considered in 'at risk' patients, particularly those in psychiatric and geriatric wards. . . ."

In a later issue of the *British Medical Journal* (May 1, 1971), a London physician reports still another case. This was a 64-year-old man with a three-week history of shortness of breath and cough. He appeared to have all the symptoms of heart failure. His lungs showed infection. He was given large doses of antibiotics. His ankles were badly swollen and the swelling did not go down. He was given several diuretics, those drugs which usually cause urination and disappearance of accumulation of water in tissues. There were no results.

Someone thought of beriberi. He was immediately given thiamine by injection. The swelling disappeared. The man lost considerable weight which had been largely unwanted water. And he was cured. The physician then asked about his diet. It seems he was a heavy drinker, ate a very poor diet and had a mild deficiency in iron. All this would indicate that he was not eating nearly enough of foods rich in thiamine. The recommended daily dietary allowances for thiamine, as released by the National Academy of Sciences in 1968, range from 0.2 milligrams for infants to 1.5 milligrams for growing teenage boys. Adults generally require from 1 to 1.4 milligrams each day. For the thiamine content of some popular foods, see the chart on page 232.

Other cases of beriberi have been reported in the *British Medical Journal.* Recently, two patients were admitted to a London hospital with the disease. Both patients were suffering from severe heart and respiratory symptoms. No one at first thought of beriberi as a possible diagnosis, of course.

The first patient was a young college student who had arrived in Britain only nine months before and was apparently living on a small budget, since his diet had been "monotonous and much of it was carbohydrate." He had severe breathlessness, weakness, pain in the chest and upper abdomen. His face and ankles were swollen. He was restless and agitated.

The doctors went to work on him and dosed him with many kinds of drugs, tested all aspects of his condition and remained puzzled. Then someone suggested beriberi. It didn't seem possible, since he did not have some of the most important symptoms of this condition, in terms of heart damage. But they gave him thiamine. Almost immediately his condition began to improve. The swelling disappeared and the breathlessness and the pounding heart righted themselves. "Over a period of several days all clinical evidence of circulatory and renal abnormality cleared," the doctors reported.

They sent him home, apparently without any advice on diet, since nothing of this sort is mentioned in the article. He didn't return for follow-up, so presumably he is back on his high carbohydrate diet which will undoubtedly produce the same condition again, as soon as he has exhausted his store of thiamine.

The second case was a 62-year-old man, breathless, swollen ankles, confusion, a poor memory. He lived alone, ate irregularly and drank a lot of beer. He also had several symptoms of scurvy, the disease of vitamin C deficiency.

The doctors gave him thiamine and vitamin C and he began to improve at once. "All abnormalities of cardiopulmonary function resolved after thiamine therapy," said the two doctors.

In their discussion of these two cases, the doctors, Neil McIntyre and Nigel N. Stanley, point out that what happened in these two patients did not show the usual symptoms of beriberi affecting the heart. Nevertheless, the B vitamin worked its miracle.

These two sensible doctors suggest, finally, that, since the treatment is completely harmless, it might be a good idea to give thiamine in any case where the patient has had heart failure without any clear evidence as to the cause! Why not indeed? And what might be even better, why not try giving all the B vitamins as well as vitamin C, A and E in large doses to all hospital patients the moment they come in the door, without waiting to diagnose, treat, or give drugs! Isn't it possible that many disorders which bring people to hospitals are the result of plain nutritional deficiency day after day and year after year?

Medical journals occasionally describe modern cases of pellagra, the disease of niacin deficiency.

Deficiency in just one vitamin is uncommon. When the diet is so unbalanced that one vitamin is missing, others are bound to be missing, too.

What kind of diet might produce beriberi or pellagra? A diet that relies almost completely on refined and processed cereals—white, unenriched bread and any of a number of popular breakfast cereals. To prevent these easily preventable disorders, one should make certain to eat enough meat, fish, poultry, eggs, milk, and green, leafy vegetables like spinach and chard. The other sources are wholegrain cereals and breads—really wholegrain.

Interestingly enough, in the early days of vitamin research when pills were not available, doctors cured cases of pellagra and beriberi with brewer's yeast, wheat germ, bran and liver. So include them in your meals as often as you can. Yeast can be added to everything you bake and every suitable dish like casseroles, soups, salads, etc. Wheat germ is great, eaten with milk and honey as a breakfast cereal. Its whopping big content of protein and minerals make it a stick-to-the-ribs breakfast equivalent to bacon and eggs. The bran which is removed from whole grains to make refined flours is available as a cereal—a food noted for its ability to preserve "regularity".

A worried Texas physician asked in the *Journal of the American Medical Association*, February 6, 1967, "What are the usual causes of burning sensations in the soles of the feet in elderly persons?"

The JAMA editor talked about muscle cramping, impaired circulation and possible diabetes—and deficiency in thiamine and pyridoxine.

Nutritional Disorders of the Nervous System, by John D. Spillane, describes the burning feet complaint of people with pellagra and prisoners of war who are given far too little of the B vitamins. Old folks have a tendency to eat foods that are easy to buy, prepare and chew—like white bread, refined cereals and sweets. This is bound to result in B vitamin deficiency.

Three Australian physicians report in the July 10, 1971 issue of *The Lancet*, a British medical journal, on a 48-year-old alcoholic patient with brain deterioration due to long years of heavy drinking. Two weeks before he came to the hospital he found he had difficulty in walking. He staggered and could not coordinate the movements of his legs. Other symptoms pointed to quite serious brain damage—the kind that heavy drinking eventually produces. He was given a richly nourishing diet and very high doses of thiamine. This was 200 milligrams by injection and 300 milligrams by mouth every day. Remember, the recommended daily allowance for a man is 1.4 milligrams daily.

So this alcoholic was getting more than 500

times the amount specified for a non-alcoholic. He was also given massive doses of riboflavin and niacin. Within about three weeks he was able to leave the hospital and was given thiamine to take in massive doses. His symptoms improved and he was able to walk almost normally. Had he been able to stay on the wagon, the physicians are sure he could have recovered completely. We will have more to say about alcholism and B vitamin therapy later in this book.

A University of Alabama medical researcher has discovered a significant relationship between the amount of thiamine in one's meals and the frequency of complaints related to heart disease and the possibility of heart attacks.

It has been known for some time, report Dr. E. Cheraskin and his colleagues, writing in the *Journal of the American Geriatrics Society* for November 1967, that there is a definite relation between the amount of carbohydrate food eaten —especially refined carbohydrate—and the frequency of these heart complaints. It is also well known, they go on, that thiamine is part of the complicated process that goes on in our bodies to change carbohydrate foods into energy.

To discover whether it's possible to relate conclusively a lack of vitamin B to tendency to heart attacks, Dr. Cheraskin asked 74 dentists and their wives to participate in a study. Each of them was asked a series of questions which we reproduce here, all having to do with heart and artery health. Then he asked each of these people to keep records of what they ate and he

TEST QUESTIONS ON HEART AND CIRCULATORY COMPLAINTS FROM THE CORNELL UNIVERSITY MEDICAL SCHOOL

1. Has a doctor ever said your blood pressure was too high?
2. Has a doctor ever said your blood pressure was too low?
3. Do you have pains in the heart or chest?
4. Are you often bothered by thumping of the heart?
5. Does your heart often race like mad?
6. Do you often have difficulty breathing?
7. Do you get out of breath long before anyone else?
8. Do you sometimes get out of breath just sitting still?
9. Are your ankles often badly swollen?
10. Do cold hands or feet trouble you even in hot weather?
11. Do you suffer from frequent cramps in your legs?
12. Has a doctor ever said you have heart trouble?
13. Does heart trouble run in your family?

checked their food intake for its content of thiamine.

He found, interestingly enough, that more than one-fourth of these folks were getting less thiamine in their meals than the officially recommended daily allowance. He then divided the dentists and their wives into two groups—those getting rather high amounts of the B vitamin, and those getting lower amounts. Then he checked on the heart and artery complaints of the two groups and found that, on an average basis for the whole group, those folks who were eating less thiamine had more heart and artery complaints than those who got more thiamine. In fact, almost twice as many had complaints in the group which got less thiamine.

Then Dr. Cheraskin reminded himself that age may have a considerable amount to do with health, since any disorder tends to become worse as we grow older and less able to withstand it. So he decided to check the age of the different people having heart complaints and compare this with the amount of thiamine in their diets. He found that the older people who ate the least thiamine had the most complaints. The younger people who ate food containing most thiamine had the fewest complaints.

But he also found that the older people who ate food containing the most thiamine had fewer heart and artery complaints than young people whose meals tended to be short on the B vitamin. He warns us that these figures do not prove beyond a shadow of a doubt that the amount of thiamine you get every day is directly related to whether or not you have circulatory trouble. He thinks that more experiments must be done in which thiamine supplements are given to many people and their circulatory problems are checked before and after the vitamin is given.

We have several further comments on what we consider is an extremely valuable piece of research. First, since it is well known that thiamine is essential for the body's use of carbohydrates—that is, starch and sugar—it seems quite likely that anyone who eats a lot of foods high in starch and sugar from which all the thiamine has been removed is bound to be lacking in this important vitamin. Thiamine accompanies starches and sugar in such foods as grains and sugarcane. There is enough thiamine in both of these natural foods to provide for all the body needs for digesting and assimilating the starches and sugars.

But when most of this thiamine is removed, as modern processors do when they refine cereals, make white flour out of whole grain flour and white sugar out of sugarcane, the folks who eat these foods are almost bound to be short on thiamine—unless they provide it in some other way.

Then, too, when we eat lots of such depleted foods as white flour and white sugar, we use up space in our menus that should be devoted to more nutritious foods. So we probably get far less thiamine in other foods, since we simply don't have room left to eat enough of these nutritious foods, stuffed as we are with refined carbohydrates.

The child or the over-weight reducer, for example, who eats some refined sugar between meals in the form of soft drinks or candy may manage to spoil his appetite for the next meal, and, at the same time, he has given his digestive apparatus a problem it can't solve—a lot of sugar or starch without the wherewithal to handle it. And, by spoiling his appetite for the next meal, he gets even less of the important nutrients which he might have gotten in meat, wholemeal bread, vegetables, nuts and seeds, etc. He just didn't have the appetite to eat them. The sugary snack spoiled it.

It seems reasonable that, the longer such a state of affairs goes on, the greater will be the strain on those parts of us that depend on thiamine for easy, successful functioning. The heart and arteries, for example. So as we grow older, the circulatory complaints increase as our shortage of thiamine increases. But note, too, that if we have continually gotten enough thiamine, according to Dr. Cheraskin's investigation, our circulatory machinery tends to stay in good order, better order, in fact, than that of younger people who are short on thiamine.

We generally think of cirrhosis of the liver as the classical disease of alcoholics. But many other conditions contribute to the ill-health of these unfortunates. *Archives of Internal Medicine* for October 1967 presented the case of a 36-year-old man suffering from heart failure and acute failure of the kidneys. He was found to be severly deficient in thiamine. So long had the deficiency been going on that his doctor thought that the man was suffering from beriberi. This man had depended on alcohol for the calories to keep himself going. He had stopped eating nourishing food.

Since pure carbohydrate, which is what alcohol is, makes heavy demands on the body's store of thiamine, it is no wonder that the patient eventually degenerated into a beriberi patient. A massive dose of thiamine brought his kidneys back to normal, suggesting that the heart condition, brought on by the lack of thiamine, had caused the kidney condition.

Never underestimate the power of the B vitamins and their essential place in your meals and food supplements.

CHAPTER 3

Riboflavin

On March 9, 1972 the Congressional authors of the new cancer-attack law introduced a $1.3 billion bill to intensify the battle against heart, lung and blood-vessel diseases. Sen. Edward Kennedy (D., Mass.) and Rep. Paul G. Rogers (D., Fla.), the co-sponsors, said that the proposed legislation was aimed at arresting diseases which annually cause more than half the deaths in the United States. Under the legislation there would be community-based centers for screening and education as part of a disease-control program. In addition, there would be 15 new clinical research and demonstration centers for cardiovascular diseases and the same number of clinical research facilities for pulmonary diseases.

In the past, too little attention has been paid to the prevention of diseases, rather than trying to cure the disease after the patient has contracted it. And there is every indication that most of our major ills may be nutritionally based. Such things as cancer, heart disease, multiple sclerosis, alcoholism, cataracts, mental disorders —yes, even aging—may be due to an imbalance of nutrients in our bodies or perhaps a damaging shortage of one or more vitamins or minerals.

Riboflavin, or vitamin B2, is only one of the substances that may turn out to be in the forefront of this fight. A yellowish nitrogenous polyhydroxy alcohol, B2 was isolated as a vitamin in 1933 by R. Kuhn, P. Gyorgy and T. Wagner-Jauregg. It occurs in considerable portions in egg white and whole eggs, milk, whey, brewers yeast, liver, whole grains and soybeans.

Dr. Otto Heinrich Warburg, a physician, two-time Nobel Laureate and a former director of the Max Planck Institute of Cell Physiology in Germany, was a pioneer in the investigation of oxidation and reduction. One of the world's leading biochemists, Warburg theorized that cancer cells produce energy by the fermentation of sugar, rather than, as often suspected, by the normal respiratory process. He further believed that the key to cancer prevention was in the protection of cellular respiration through the utilization of riboflavin and niacin. Dr. Warburg, who died in August 1970 at the age of 86, was also one of the first to discover the high production of lactic acid (an acid found in the blood and connected with muscle fatigue) by cancer tissues. Hopefully, other researchers are continuing Dr. Warburg's important research.

Dr. Albert B. Sabin, developer of the oral polio vaccine that bears his name, told the Fifth International Symposium on Comparative Leukemia Research at Padua, Italy in 1971, that more research is needed on the role of nutrition in the possible prevention of cancer. He told the congress that crash programs to develop a miraculous cancer vaccine cure, rather than a method of prevention, are doomed to failure.

We usually think of anemia having to do with a lack of iron in food. And there is more serious anemia caused by certain very toxic drugs. As we learn from the medical journals, pernicious anemia can be prevented and cured by taking vitamin B12, along with certain substances that help the stomach to absorb it. According to two Baylor University researchers in Texas, however, a deficiency of riboflavin can cause anemia. Eight volunteers were put on a diet from which all riboflavin was carefully excluded. Then they were given vitamin supplements to make sure that they had enough of all other vitamins and minerals. The volunteers rapidly developed anemia, resulting in disorders of the blood cells and of the bone marrow where certain blood cells are manufactured. When vitamin B2 was given again, the anemia was halted.

Cataract, which is generally thought to be a disorder of old age, affects over five million Americans between the ages of 30 and 60. Cataract is a fogging of the eye lens and may eventually result in complete blindness. The medical treatment is an operation which removes the cataract; then special glasses are prescribed. Unfortunately, many of the operations are not successful.

Cataract can easily be produced in laboratory animals by depriving them of riboflavin. In one experiment all the rats whose diets contained no vitamin B2 got cataract. But it was only early in life that the deficient diet produced the effect—in other words, the rats were young when they got the diet that was lacking in the B vitamin.

Guinea pigs and man are just a few of the animals which cannot manufacture their own vitamin C. So diets deficient in vitamin C can produce scurvy. These same diets can also produce cataracts. A diet low in protein has also been linked to this eye disorder.

Adelle Davis, who has written many excellent books, including *Let's Get Well,* stated: "My files contain dozens of unsolicited letters from persons who have recovered from cataracts after their diets were more adequate, often while they were preparing for surgery. People sometimes take only a riboflavin supplement and then wonder why their eyes fail to improve. An antistress diet high in protein, riboflavin, vitamin C, vitamin E, pantothenic acid and all nutrients is essential before good results can be expected." (Additional information on the relationship between cataracts and nutrition is published in *Vitamin C, the Powerhouse Vitamin, Conquers More Than Just Colds,* which is listed in the bibliography at the end of this book).

Four important studies of aging people seem to demonstrate two related facts: 1. Lack of essential nutrients may be a very common cause of aging; and 2. Older folks may in truth be getfar less than they need of many essential food elements.

Geriatrics for March 1968 published an article by three Chicago researchers on the actual circumstances of our approximately 20 million senior citizens where eating and nutrition are concerned. They asked questions about the kind of diet being eaten by the elderly and the reasons for it. Their conclusions are significant.

First, they point out that, although babies differ greatly in their individual physiological make-up, old folks differ far more, since they have a lifetime to accumulate all kinds of damage from accidents, surgery, disease, poisons from drugs and pollution, along with bad habits such as smoking and eating unwisely. So, if we agree that each of us is different in his needs, we must go farther with older folks and decide that each of them is even more varied from all other old folks in his present condition and needs.

Then, too, we must admit that most old folks suffer from at least one chronic disorder. According to these scientists, about 75% of all people between 65 and 74 years of age have chronic conditions and the incidence is even higher in those over 75. And, as we learned at the White House Conference on Aging in 1971, disease is not the only problem our senior citizens face. Lack of money and means of transportation, loneliness and inadequate nutrition are some of the others.

A 1955 dietary survey revealed that homes with homemakers over 60 and older have poorer diets in regard to all nutrients than households with younger cooks. Riboflavin, calcium and vitamin C were the essentials most often lacking. Iron and thiamine are also usually in short supply. As people age beyond 65, their diets become progressively worse. Tea, toast, cereals and sweets are most often favored. Some of the results of such badly planned diets are widespread anemia due to lack of iron and a bone condition that is almost universal—osteoporosis—which many nutrition experts believe is caused chiefly by lack of calcium and vitamin D.

Since obesity and overweight are rather common among old folks, it seems apparent that the day's calories which should be spent in high protein foods (rich in vitamins and minerals) are often wasted instead on non-nourishing foods which contribute little but excess weight. Those on reducing diets tend to lack vitamins and minerals, since it is hard to plan such diets which will supply all the needed nutrients.

The conclusion these authors came to was that perhaps one-third or more of all people 65 and over have diets containing less than the recommended amounts of essential nutrients, especially vitamin B2, vitamin C and calcium.

Another study, made by six physicians at a British hospital catering only to old people, was published in *Gerontologica Clinica* (Volume 10, 1968). They examined 80 elderly patients who had lived in the hospital for a long time. They looked for signs of vitamin deficiency in the majority of patients. Only seven of the 80 appeared to be relatively free of such symptoms.

To make sure that the symptoms indicated vitamin deficiency and nothing else, they divided the group into two groups and gave one group a vitamin supplement, the other a simple pill which contained nothing. The group getting the vitamin supplement showed improvement within six months, much more improvement within a year. The group which received no vitamin supplement showed no improvement. Especially interesting was the fact that apparently unrelated symptoms—like bed sores—yielded to the vitamin supplement.

Said the authors: "One feature that has been observed in this study is the slow rate at which certain of the pathological (disease) changes can be reversed by even high doses of vitamins. It would seem that, like many other conditions, early changes are reversible but that if these remain untreated for a sufficient length of time then irreversible changes occur."

In a third article bearing on this subject, three Connecticut doctors studied 50 men and women at a nursing home for the aged trying to discover whether they suffered from being unable to absorb the food they ate. These older folks suffered from what the doctors called "The usual diseases of old age, such as osteoporosis, arteriosclerosis (hardening of the arteries), general mental confusion and so forth." Nine of them showed symptoms of severe wasting. That is, they were excessively thin, apathetic and suffering from severe mental abnormalities.

Is it possible, the doctors asked in this study, that one reason for the condition of these old people is just that they do not absorb enough nutrients from their food to bring them good health? They found that this, indeed, was the case. Many of the patients were unable to absorb important essential nutrients like protein, vitamin A, fat (which influences the absorption of all fat-soluble vitamins—A, D, E and K).

The investigators also found that all of them were suffering, to some degree, from an inability to handle starches and sugars. That is, their blood sugar levels were disordered. They tended toward being diabetic. The patients who appeared to be wasting away were found to be least able to absorb their food properly.

The fourth article that we refer to appeared in the April 1966 issue of the *Journal of the American Geriatrics Society*. Written by a Belgian physician, a specialist in the problems of older people, it takes the form of a new theory on why we age. No one really knows, of course, just why or how we get old or why some people seem to age so much faster than others.

Piecing together information from many different sources, Dr. H. LeComte presented his new theory of aging: that we age because we have serious deficiencies in essential nutrients. Severe premature aging is caused by serious deficiencies; less pronounced aging is caused by lesser deficiencies and so on. "From this we conclude that the so-called 'normal aging' is caused by small (maybe not to be diagnosed, but, nevertheless, real) deficiencies," he said.

He tells us that the illness or illnesses of an elderly patient can be far more easily cured if he is amply supplied with all the things in which he has been deficient. Then he tells us that there is a large group of older folks who appear to be healthy but who complain of "all sorts of troubles of which fatigue is the most important." These complaints, he said, are the results of one or several deficiencies and they can be treated by supplying the essential nutrients in plentiful amounts. (Another theory on why we grow old is explored in the book, *Vitamin E, Wonder Worker of the '70's?*", listed in the bibliography).

In order to determine how much of each vitamin and mineral we need each day, every household should have a copy of *Recommended Dietary Allowances,* 7th Edition, 1968, available from the Printing and Publishing Office, National Academy of Sciences, 2101 Constitution Ave., Washington, D. C. 20418. It costs $1.75. The next edition is due out in 1973.

For example, how much riboflavin do you need each day? For infants, the official daily recommendation is from 0.4 to 0.6 milligrams; for children, from 0.6 to 1.2 milligrams; for males, its 1.3 for boys up to 1.7 for adults; for women, the range is 1.3 milligrams for girls to 1.5 milligrams for adults; pregnancy requires 1.8 milligrams daily and for lactation 2 milligrams each day. A chart on page 234 gives some of the major sources of riboflavin.

CHAPTER 4

Niacin

A NO MORE dramatic disease has ever come to the medical profession than pellagra, according to Dr. Tom Spies, one of the world's greatest medical authorities in the field of nutrition. Pellagra has been known throughout the world for centuries, yet, it was not until the early 1930's that Dr. Spies and several others managed to cure severely ill pellagra patients.

The cure was a simple one: enormous doses of brewer's yeast, combined with a diet "high in calories, protein, minerals and vitamins." By 1935, Dr. Spies had found that the one ounce of brewer's yeast he had been giving was not enough, and, when he doubled and tripled this amount, cure was almost miraculous.

The symptoms of pellagra are a red, sore

tongue, skin troubles, digestive troubles, along with diarrhea and nerve disorders so severe that patients may become insane. Said Dr. Spies: "No tissues of the body are entirely exempt if the disease is permitted to run its natural course, untreated."

Pellagra can be induced in laboratory animals by giving them a diet deficient in niacin. It can also be induced by giving them a diet consisting largely of corn products, because corn, although it is an excellent food in other respects, is deficient in one amino acid (tryptophan) and niacin. Although this does no harm in a diet including other protein-rich foods, someone who is living mostly on foods made from corn is risking pellagra. The disease was widespread during the depression of the 1930's in the southern part of the U.S., where corn bread, hominy, grits and other corn products formed a large part of the diet.

Dr. Spies writes in *Clinical Nutrition*, that there are three groups of people who are most likely to be susceptible to pellagra. First, those who do not eat a nourishing diet, either because they do not have enough money to buy nourishing foods, because they do not know which foods to eat or because they have peculiar notions about food and put themselves on diets that are deficient in the B vitamins.

The second group consists of those who have

organic diseases which have changed their eating habits or have made their needs for certain foods much greater. People with tuberculosis, diseases of the digestive tract, cirrhosis of the liver, heart disease, certain kinds of kidney disease, diabetes, amoebic dysentery, pneumonia, hookworm, influenza, typhoid fever, malaria and other diseases interfering with the eating of foods containing the B vitamins and the absorption of these vitamins from foods.

The third group are chronic alcoholics who neglect all food and try to live on alcohol.

Often the sufferer from pellagra is piteously thin and starved-looking. But it is just as likely that he is overweight, for, if he is eating a diet high in refined carbohydrates and fats, he is not getting enough of the B vitamins to protect him from pellagra, although he may be getting enough calories to make him fat.

Many modern American mothers who make little effort to study nutrition and allow their children to live on soft drinks, potato chips and candy are guaranteeing a future for these children in which they will be threatened with pellagra—if they manage to escape such diseases as TB, diabetes and heart trouble. Mothers and children must be made aware of the overwhelming importance of foods high in protein, vitamins and minerals.

How can you cure pellagra? In the words of

Dr. Tom Spies: "113 grams of wheat germ daily (about one-fourth pound), 57 grams of bewer's yeast daily (about 4 tablespoons) or a concentrate of niacin which would, of course, have to be given by a physician." In cases where the patient cannot absorb food effectively from his digestive tract, the B vitamin can be injected.

Unfortunately, pellagra did not pass into oblivion in the 1930s. It is still very much with us in the 1970s. A headline in the *Washington Post* for April 2, 1971 read: "Mental patients hit by pellagra." The article went on to say that "Maryland's health chief said that he personally discovered in December that patients at state mental hospitals were receiving inadequate daily amounts of vitamins in their meals, causing many of them to contract pellagra. The deficiencies apparently had existed for years and years," stated Dr. Neil Solomon.

The patients were immediately given vitamins, but Dr. Solomon explained that, because of budget cutting, there would not be enough money to feed mental patients properly during the coming years. There were, at the time, 10,-300 patients in mental hospitals in the state.

Dr. Solomon, a specialist in nutrition, said he had noticed a tremendous number of patients "had red, swollen tongues and lesions (sores) on exposed parts of their bodies." The hospital attendants—and presumably all the doctors and psychiatrists in attendance—had not noticed anything wrong with the patients, the *Post* article continued.

When Dr. Solomon visited the hospital kitchens and studied the menus, he found that meals were deficient not only in niacin, but also protein, iron and calcium. "An unspecified number of patients had pellagra," he noted. He went on to say that he had no idea how many mental patients had gotten pellagra in the past or how many had died of it. The same could be said for other deficiency diseases. The state had been spending 72 cents per day per patient to feed the mentally ill in six institutions. An additional 28 cents per day had brought the menus to at least a nutritionally sound basis.

Dr. Solomon is, apparently, just one of a handful of doctors in the entire medical profession who is concerned about what patients eat. Speaking at a symposium on hunger and malnutrition sponsored by the American Association for the Advancement of Science, Dr. Jean Mayer, professor of Nutrition at Harvard University, and President Nixon's advisor on nutrition, said:

"Our studies at Harvard among residents suggests that the average physician knows a little more about nutrition than the average secretary—unless the secretary has a weight problem, and then she probably knows more than the average physician." He said that only a half dozen or so medical schools in the country include a nutrition course for their students.

Continued Dr. Mayer: "Nutrition education should be centered on foods—their size, shape, color, caloric value, etc. We must relate such vital information to the everyday uses of people."

In 1963, the Council on Foods and Nutrition of the American Medical Association issued a report on nutritional education in medical schools in which they opined that the medics were not really learning anything much about food and nutrition, and they suggested hiring one professor in each school whose main interest might be nutrition. Even Dr. Fredrick Stare of Harvard, writing in *Nutrition Reviews*, said that very little attention is directed to nutrition teaching in medical schools. In the *American Journal of Public Health* for June 1966, Dr. Robert Shank stated that the situation is very bad. In 1967, Dr. J. F. Mueller said that there is great dissatisfaction among nutritionists in general with "the quality of nutrition education in medical schools." Dr. Robert H. Barnes of the University of Washington, concurred. Writing in *Nutrition Today*, 1968, Dr. Barnes, after studying what went on in a local hospital, said that he found that the terms in which doctors order diets for their patients are completely meaningless and indicate that the doctors have no idea of what the diets are supposed to do for the patients or why they should be put on such diets.

Said Dr. Barnes: "No portion of the human body seems to confound physicians more than the gastrointestinal tract. Writing a diet for a patient ailing in this dark and mysterious region seems to fill us with bewilderment."

Cancer researchers have often used vitamins A, C and E in their search for a cure for this mysterious disorder. We now have a report from the University of California at Los Angeles, where six researchers have determined that the abnormal growth of cancer cells may be due to a lack of niacin. Dr. Robert A. Smith and his co-workers have not as yet used animals or humans in their research, however, they indicate that animal studies will be begun. Working in tissue culture with cells derived from colon and kidney cancers in humans, the UCLA team found that there is a marked difference between cancerous and normal cells. The cancer cells were depleted of nicotinamide, the physiologically active form of niacin, they said.

A Montreal, Canada professor believes that niacin is important for improving memory in aging people. He also gave them carbon dioxide to inhale. He is quoted in *Science News* for April 9, 1966 as saying that impairment of the manufacture of new protein in the body may be responsible for badly functioning memories. And the B vitamin may help to encourage this activity.

In another vein, Dr. Grace A. Goldsmith of Tulane University reported in the *Journal of the American Medical Association* for October 11, 1965 that niacin appears to reduce the level of cholesterol in the blood. In experiments with rabbits, the B vitamin protected against hardening of the arteries and reduced its severity.*

Two New York physicians, who treated 41 patients with large doses of niacin, reported similar results with respect to cholesterol. The patients were suffering from high levels of cholesterol in the blood and hardening of the arteries. In all cases, the large doses of niacin brought about a reduction in cholesterol without any change in diet. If you are bothered by large amounts of cholesterol deposits, why not ask your doctor to investigate the use of niacin? Taking an isolated B vitamin on your own in large quantities sometimes produces slight side effects because it is being used as a drug.

Idiopathic hypogeusia is the unlikely name given to a new condition the doctors have recently uncovered. It means the inability to taste anything. Several articles in medical journals have reported on this disorder, and they are mystified as to what could possibly cause such a

* Hoffer, Altchule and Stephen first reported this observation (*Archives of Biochemistry and Biophysics*, 1955).

condition. In a letter to the editor of the *Journal of the American Medical Association*, Dr. R. F. Green of Saskatchewan, Canada announced that the condition is "part of a very old disease which causes the perception to change—perceptual dysfunction, as a result of a niacin deficiency." The disease produced is pellagra and "the cure is niacin."

Dr. Green goes on to point out that lack of taste is only one possible effect on sensation caused by a lack of this B vitamin. In his experience with 300 cases, impairment of the senses of taste and smell are problems, he said. He told his physician readers that many patients come to a doctor with complaints for which there seems to be no physical basis. Ask them questions about their sense of taste, smell, sight, hearing and touch and you can diagnose the disorder, he said. He gives his patients a perceptual test which reveals their impairment of one sense or another. Then he suggests a diet, including plenty of niacin. "The results in cases of recent onset are nothing short of miraculous," he said. "Patients whose aberrations have extended over months and even years respond more slowly but yet very satisfactorily in the main."

Laboratories used to report considerable work with animals on the effects of vitamin dosages on the symptoms of old age. But this kind of research has rather gone out of style, especially since our official scientific bodies make pronouncements that old people need no more vitamins than younger folks, and taking more vitamins than you "need" will do nothing for health.

We are, therefore, glad to find in a European scientific journal the account of some convincing research along these lines. The scientists used three groups of rats and placed all of them on thc same diet. Then they gave the first group a vitamin preparation containing twice the minimum daily requirements for rats. The second group received only niacin. The third group got no vitamins at all. However, all these rats were eating the customary good, nourishing diet that is fed to valuable laboratory animals to maintain the best possible health.

The first group of animals showed better food assimilation, better health and growth than the rest of the rats. The first group and the group that got the B vitamin were more active physically than the others. The first group had higher fertility rate and lowest blood cholesterol. Those which received the multiple-vitamin had the longest lifespan. Next came those which got only the niacin, while the rats which had no vitamin supplement had the shortest life span. After the animals died, their tissues were examined in the laboratory. Deposits in the blood vessels—the kind that lead to hardening of the arteries—were much less noticeable in the rats that got the vitamin supplement. Other organs, too, showed less degeneration than that of the non-supplement animals.

To test their findings still further, the scientists gave a multiple-vitamin preparation to a group of 65- to 90-year-old people for a month. They report that, when the oldsters were tested, they showed an increase in oxidative processes and protein metabolism. There was also "improvement in their general condition," even though 30 days is not a very long time for such a study. This research was reported by V. V. Efremov in the journal *Vestnil Akademii Meditsinskikh Nauk, USSR*, Volume 21 (10), 1966. It was abstracted in *Chemical Abstracts*, 1968, on page 9111.

As far back as 1925, J. Goldberger had determined that pellagra is a deficiency disease. In 1937, C. A. Elvehjem and his associates discovered that nicotinic acid (niacin) is involved with preventing the disease.

In the chart on page 236, we give you the main sources of niacin in the human diet. As to the recommended dietary allowances they are: infants (5 to 8 mg. daily); children (8 to 15 mg. daily; males (17 to 20 mg. daily); females (13 to 15 mg. daily). pregnant women (15 mg. daily); lactation (20 mg. daily).

CHAPTER 5

Niacin and Mental Illnesses

TODAY ABOUT ONE in every 12 American adults uses tranquilizers regularly. And an estimated 17 million Americans—in and out of hospitals—are suffering from mental illness. In other words, about one out of every 10. A 1962 survey of New Yorkers demonstrated that only one out of every five is mentally well. One out of four is so disturbed as to be impaired in his social relations.

Generally speaking, doctors involved in treating mental diseases consider them entirely psychological—that is, caused by difficulties in family adjustment and jobs, feelings of insecurity and inferiority and persecution complexes. Although they use some of the same therapy favored by these men, doctors who believe in the approach of the Huxley Institute for Biosocial Research (formerly the American Schizophrenia Association) in New York think that these mental lapses, especially schizophrenia, are entirely physical in origin.

In the face of such a vast problem, it is encouraging to know that scientists are looking more deeply into the biological reasons for mental illness. Although it is fully recognized that many different emotional and environmental stresses can and do produce nervousness, strain and tension, it now seems apparent that schizophrenia may be partially caused by something in the physical make-up of the individual.

There may be, for instance, an excess of a normally occurring chemical or chemicals. There may be a deficiency of one or more of these chemicals. There may also be an accumulation of abnormal waste products in the body cells. Consequently, the body may be unable to detoxify or render harmless some naturally occurring but potentially harmful material. Mental illness, therefore, may represent a large-scale disordering of entire working systems of the body.

We know, for example, that some children are born with an inability to use certain proteins. If this inadequacy is not discovered during the first weeks of life and a special diet is not provided for the infant, such extensive damage can be done to the brain cells that the child will be mentally defective. We know, too, that injecting blood taken from patients ill with the most serious mental disorders can cause brief episodes of mental illness in perfectly healthy people and even in animals and insects.

One substance, isolated from the blood of schizophrenics and injected into a spider, will cause the spider to lose its ability to spin webs. Substances in the spider's nerves and brain which govern its ability to spin webs according to certain patterns are apparently destroyed or inactivated. The patterns become aimless, unfinished, inept. The spider, in effect, has become mentally ill.

As long ago as 1966, a newspaper headline told how a researcher at the New Jersey Neuropsychiatric Institute had used a form of niacin in treating 1,000 patients with schizophrenia. Furthermore, Dr. Humphrey Osmond said on April 4, 1966 that 75% of the patients were *cured.* This is an astonishing word to use in regard to this terrible mental illness that afflicts most of the patients in our mental hospitals. He mentioned one patient who had been ill for 29 years and was free of symptoms after only five days of treatment.

Dr. Abram Hoffer, of the Department of Public Health of Saskatchewan, Canada, formerly with the New Jersey psychiatrist, has been reporting in medical journals for about 20 years on his almost miraculous results with many patients. Some of them needed treatment over a period of many years. Dr. Hoffer was using a different form of niacin. Now, apparently, the new compound gets results in less time.

We are reminded of the case of a truck driver who was in such bad shape that he was completely unable to care for himself, and was withdrawn into silence and depression. Tranquilizers in large doses resulted in a much worsened condition. The man had hallucinations, became incontinent and delirious. Then he was given a high protein diet along with mutiple vitamins, including 150 milligrams of niacin a day. The recommended daily allowance for a man is from 14 to 20 milligrams daily. Within five days his symptoms disappeared and he was able to return home and take up a normal life. Three months later the doctor said his condition continued to improve.

It is not known how niacin brings about these astonishing results. The theory of Drs. Osmond and Hoffer is that schizophrenia is caused by a by-product of the adrenal gland, adrenochrome, which builds up in the body and produces the hallucinations, the mania, the depression and other frightening disturbances involved in this disorder. Supposedly, different forms of niacin have the power of preventing this buildup and hence maintaining a normal mental health.

Said Dr. Hoffer, in an article published in *Lancet*, February 10, 1962: "Niacin has some though not all the qualities of an ideal treatment; it is safe, cheap and easy to administer and it uses a known pharmaceutical substance which can be taken for years on end if necessary . . . Why then have these benefits passed almost unheeded? (One reason) may be the extraordinary proliferation of the phenothiazine derivatives since 1954. (These are tranquilizers). Unlike these, niacin is a simple, well known vitamin which can be bought cheaply in bulk and cannot be patented, and there has been no campaign to persuade doctors of its usefulness."

The two doctors go into greater detail about their theories in their book, *How to Live with Schizophrenia*, published by University Books, New Hyde Park, N. Y.

"Schizophrenia is a common disease which affects the whole body, and the only mystery is that many people are still unable to recognize it as such," the doctors explain. "When you have schizophrenia you are actually physically ill, but the symptoms are both physical and mental for the disease has a specific effect on the brain. You may be fatigued, listless or depressed. Your skin may change to a darker hue, and your skin and your muscle tone may not be as good as it once was. Your eyes may have a glazed unnatural look. You will find the chief changes occurring in the way you see, think, feel and act . . ."

The remarkable thing about the theory is that the two vitamins that they use—niacin and vitamin C—can, over a period of time, repair the damaged mechanism in the mentally ill person's body and bring him back to good health. Both are used in extremely large doses as if they were drugs, rather than just food elements. The authors explain in their book that they have found a certain substance in the urine of schizophrenics which is absent from that of normal folks. Going farther into the subject in many years of laboratory experiments and experiments on themselves, they have traced the exact succession of events that takes place in the body of the ill person and the step at which something goes awry. Then they decided to try to prevent this step.

One of the reasons why their treatment isn't more widely accepted is that it does not work quickly. It may take several weeks or months to achieve its beneficial results. It may have to be prescribed for years. Also, "very few studies of this kind are made in psychiatry because they are so expensive." Drs. Hoffer and Osmond explain that there is an impression that doses of niacin this large may be harmful. This is just not true, they say, and they add that, in other experiments, very large doses have been given in successful attempts to lower cholesterol in the blood. No harmful effects have ever been seen, they added.

In addition to the niacin, they give their patients three grams of vitamin C daily until they are well. This is 3,000 milligrams. The daily recommended dosage for healthy adults is 55 milligrams for women and 60 milligrams for men. Both vitamin C and the B Complex are water-soluble vitamins, meaning that most of them pass out of the body three or four times a day.

As Drs. Osmond and Hoffer delved deeper into the subject, they reasoned that, if something went wrong with adrenalin metabolism, another substance might be produced instead which would create the terror, the mania, the distorted thinking, the delusions of persecution and the other symptoms of schizophrenia. These mental disorders—a real dementia—are the same symptoms that cropped up in the 1930's with the pellagra victims that we have already mentioned.

When they gave massive doses of niacin, they found that it benefited their patients enormously. Improvement slowed down when patients stopped taking the B vitamin. When the patients took the niacin again, they began to improve. The doctors tested large numbers of patients and followed their progress for many years, and they discovered that those taking niacin regularly showed much greater improvement than those taking no vitamin B.

British and New Zealand psychiatrists have been giving mental patients vitamin C in massive doses with excellent results. Once again, the scientific reasoning behind this is complicated. It seems that the blood of mentally disturbed patients contains a relatively large amount of copper. Copper destroys vitamin C. So the mental patient has a much greater than normal need for vitamin C. This same research, incidentally, is reported in Chapter 5 of *Vitamin C, the Powerhouse Vitamin, Conquers More Than Just Colds.*

Although we do not yet understand the many functions of the B vitamins and vitamin C in the body, we do know that stress, pollution, smoking, etc., deplete our supply of vitamin C, even though we may be getting a sufficient amount in our diet. As for the B vitamins, we have already discussed how they are removed wholesale from white flour and refined cereal products. At the same time, the body's need for them is increased, as our consumption of white sugar increases. Pellagra is caused directly by lack of niacin. Could not the more complicated but just as terrible modern forms of mental illness be caused by the lack of other B vitamins in combination with an increased need for these very vitamins?

Writing in the August 1956 issue of the *American Journal of Digestive Diseases,* Dr. Douglass

Gordon Campbell said: "No other organ of the human body is so involved with all phases of nutrition as the nervous system." This system has its own nutritional requirements. If these are not met, reversible or irreversible damage will be done to its own structure and function. It has been his experience that the great majority of mentally ill patients show signs of malnutrition. He added that the prescription of a "well-balanced diet", even if it is supplemented by vitamins and minerals, will be ineffective unless this good diet is absorbed properly by the body. Therefore, conditions must be provided for this, too.

"Unfortunately," Dr. Campbell said, "'neurologists and psychiatrists have, in the main, been too much influenced by the verbally defined limits of their specialties to pay sufficient attention to the nutriture of their patients. . . . We know that the nervous system is predominantly dependent upon blood sugar and oxygen. Deficiencies of either lead to a wide spectrum of clinical disorders," Dr. Campbell continued.

Doctors who are nutritionally oriented know the importance of maintaining correct blood sugar levels. Too high, they result in diabetes. Too low, they bring hypoglycemia (low blood sugar), with its nervousness, dizziness, fatigue, possible blackouts and other serious disorders. Consequently, more doctors are beginning to realize that these diseases—perhaps like many other diseases—may be caused by a simple malnutrition or unbalanced mealtime eating, and the realization that they can be prevented and treated by a nourishing diet with added supplements to make up for individual needs that may be excessively high, or for individual ways of life that bring about demands for far more protein, vitamins and minerals than even the average "good diet" can provide. Likely candidates for malnutrition, schizophrenia, etc., would seem to be the millions of people who go on crash reducing diets that are not supervised by a physician. Such a diet is bound to be nutritionally inadequate.

A more recent book is *New Hope for Incurable Diseases* by Dr. E. Cheraskin and Dr. W. M. Ringsdorf, Jr., of the University of Alabama. It is an excellent book for every health seeker, containing an especially fine chapter on the treatment of schizophrenia. In other chapters, the authors explore the possible causes of multiple sclerosis, glaucoma, alcoholism, aging, etc.

A Baylor University psychiatrist has cured a schizophrenic patient with a high protein diet and multiple vitamins, which included 150 milligrams of niacin. The story, which appeared in the *American Journal of Psychiatry*, is considered astonishing because, according to *Drug Trade News* for August 30, 1965, although chronic brain syndrome (disorder) associated with a vitamin deficiency is a fairly common condition, "acute brain syndrome associated with avitaminosis (vitamin deficiency) is relatively rare."

This particular patient had suffered from inability to work, loss of interest in surroundings, loss of appetite, food allergies, dizziness, fainting spells, headaches, shortness of breath and nervousness for over 20 years. According to the psychiatrist, these symptoms disappeared after five days on the high-protein, high-vitamin diet, and, three months later, the patient was free of all symptoms and leading a well-adjusted life.

Subclinical pellagra is the term that Dr. Glen Green uses in a speech reproduced in the newsletter of the then named American Schizophrenia Association for July 1970. He describes the symptoms in one 10-year-old girl who was a patient of his. Once bright, interested and alert, she began to complain of abdominal pains and headaches. Once an excellent student, she was now getting poor grades. She was cranky, refused to play the piano, once her joy.

Dr. Green examined her and could find no physical symptoms which might be causing her troubles. He then began with what he calls "perceptual" symptoms. He asked what words on a blackboard look like. She told him they wriggle around and move back and forth. There is a fog between her eyes and the blackboard. When she looks in the mirror her face becomes bigger, then smaller. Other peoples' faces seem to do the same. The ground moves beneath her feet and buildings appear to be falling on her. She sometimes feels she is not really walking on the ground. She hears voices calling her name. She is afraid of the dark, afraid of school, unhappy and depressed.

Dr. Green started her on niacin, giving her enormous doses of it—1 gram three times a day. This is almost 3,000 times the official recommended daily amount. It was given in three doses because, as we mentioned, the B vitamins are water soluble, hence are excreted rapidly, so to keep the body tissues saturated they should be taken frequently.

Within two weeks she was greatly improved but still had some complaints. By the end of a month she was completely cured and had returned to being her former happy, bright, alert self. Dr. Green says he has treated as many as 200 patients suffering from this disorder. They notice first that they are tired without reason. They are afraid without reason. They are frightened, depressed and they sleep poorly. They come to the doctor with these physical complaints because they know they need help. He examines them and can usually find nothing wrong.

But Dr. Green continues the examination. He asks the patient about perceptual changes. Do things look peculiar or taste bad? Does he have peculiar sensations while walking or lying down? Do things get suddenly big, then little again? He finds, he reports, that about 10% of the people who come to him have these troubles, which can be cured almost miraculously by massive doses of niacin.

The sooner the disease is diagnosed, the sooner it can be cured. The less protein in their diets, the greater the chance the disease will appear. It tends to run in families. If the patient has had the symptoms for only a few weeks, he can be cured in a few days.

Dr. Green calls this disorder "subclinical pellagra" for several reasons. First, its symptoms are similar to those of pellagra. Although the perceptual symptoms are those of schizophrenia, parents don't want to hear that their children are suffering from this terrible affliction. "Subclinical pellagra" sounds a little better. He adds that many inmates in the penitentiary have the disorder and he thinks they are there *because* they have it. Children who wet the bed, who do poorly in school, who can't see the blackboard in class, who sleep poorly can very often be greatly benefited by taking these large amounts of niacin and following the recommended diet.

Then he said: "Many teenagers have (subclinical pellagra) but many will not accept treatment. I feel that many of these children are the ones who take pot and LSD trying to find out what is wrong with them."

Dr. Linus Pauling believes that malnutrition in just one part of the body, the brain and nervous system whose nutritional requirements are very high, can cause mental illness. It is his contention that an individual may have no other symptoms of scurvy or pellagra and still have brain cells which suffer from impairment as a result of not enough vitamin B and vitamin C. Writing in the April 19, 1968 issue of *Science*, Dr. Pauling, twice winner of the Nobel Prize, stated that the proper functioning of the brain requires the presence of many different substances. Among these are the B Complex, vitaman C and certain protein substances. It is also true, he continued, that mental disease, usually combined with physical symptoms, results from a low concentration of these substances in the brain.

Addressing the 2nd International Congress of Social Psychiatry in London in 1969, Dr. Pauling said that he and his colleague, Dr. Arthur B. Robinson, had found an abnormally low level of vitamin C in the body fluids of about one-third of the schizophrenics they had examined.

There is now a growing recognition that the hyperactive "problem" child, the child with a learning disability and the one that causes his teachers and principal undue concern, may be suffering from a physical disorder related chiefly to nutrition and the possibly very high nutritional requirements of some of these children. This is the viewpoint of Dr. Allan Cott, a private psychiatrist who practices in New York.

Dr. Cott enlarged on this theory in an article in *Schizophrenia*, Volume 3, Number 2. The title of the article is "Orthomolecular Approach to the Treatment of Learning Disabilities." "Orthomolecular" is a word first used by Dr. Linus Pauling several years ago, when he proposed his world-shaking theory that we mentioned a few pages back. The victim may not appear to be suffering from malnutrition for he may have no other symptoms of vitamin or mineral deficiency. Yet, there may be malnutrition in parts of the brain and nervous system.

Dr. Cott and many other psychiatrists and physicians are at present treating patients with this theory as the basis for their work. They are using massive doses of a number of vitamins, in the belief that these patients have extra large requirements for these vitamins. Many of the physicians use a special diet as well.

In his article, Dr. Cott reported that, in the last five years, he has treated 500 children with this approach and has had better results than he has had with any other kind of treatment. He said there are very few cases of dramatic response by disturbed children treated with the usual drugs. You will remember that, in 1971, there were disclosures that in many public schools "difficult" and "hyperactive" children are being treated with drugs by the school physicians. The wisdom of this method was questioned by many people. Now Dr. Cott tells us that the response of the children is poor.

He believes in using megadoses of a number of vitamins—not just one or two. He said that up to 1,000 times the usual vitamin doses may be required. He has successfully treated adults with massive doses of niacin, pyridoxine, C, E and others. He has had remarkable results in treating schizophrenia. So he began treatment of schizophrenic and autistic (daydreaming) children and "found improvement in many of these children to be more dramatic than in adults." He further stated that the treatment is most effective if it is given to difficult children when they are quite young. As they grow older, longer and longer treatment is needed.

Dr. Cott's descriptions of these unfortunate children are arresting. He said that, in most instances, within three to six months the child begins to understand and obey commands. He shows a willingness to cooperate with parents and teachers. The hyperactivity—which is one of the main symptoms of the childhood mental troubles—begins to subside.

These children who are brought to him have been exposed to "every form of treatment and every known tranquilizer and sedative with little or no success, even in controlling the hyperactivity." After treatment with massive vitamin therapy, those who have never spoken begin to babble. Those who can already speak begin to show steady improvement in forming phrases and short sentences. "In their general behavior, they show a greater appreciation for the people in their environment," Dr. Cott said. "They become more loving and not only permit cuddling and hugging, but seek it. Bizarre food choices change slowly to include a larger variety of foods."

Dr. Cott gives disturbed children and children with learning disabilities these vitamins: Niacin or niacinamide (another form of this B vitamin)—one to two grams daily, depending on weight. Vitamin C—one to two grams daily. Pyridoxine—200 to 400 milligrams daily. Calcium pantothenate (this is one form of pantothenic acid)—400 to 600 milligrams daily. These are startling doses for little ones weighing 35 pounds or more, he said. He varies the dose depending on individual response.

Dr. Cott tells us that, in the USSR, doctors are also using vitamin B15 (pangamic acid) in cases of retardation. They believe it helps supply oxygen to brain tissues. Other miracles being wrought by simple vitamin therapy seem almost unbelievable. Dr. Cott reports on a brain-injured child who had had seizures every day for three years. Eleven days after he started on pyridoxine therapy, he had his first day free from seizures. During all those years, he had been taking the tranquilizers usually prescribed for this condition and the seizures had not stopped.

Another child who had multiple daily seizures for two years became free from seizures 72 hours after the massive doses of vitamins were begun. He was still well four years later! "I have seen very few cases of childhood schizophrenia, autism or brain injury in whom seizure activity did not respond to the megavitamins," Dr. Cott explained. Parents bringing their children for this treatment and watching their steady improvement are also cheered by realizing that the injury to the child was nutritional and biochemical in origin and was not caused by something the parent had done or neglected to do. Parents of these children so often carry enormous loads of guilt, which psychotherapy has often made heavier.

This is perhaps the most significant statement that Dr. Cott makes about diet: "The universal observations on the dietary habits of brain-injured children, hyperactive children, learning-disabled children and psychotic children have been that these children eat a diet which is high in cereals, in carbohydrate foods and those foods prepared with sugar."

He has carefully studied the blood sugar levels of this group of patients, and he has found an abnormally high incidence of low blood sugar and lack of enough insulin to handle carbohydrates properly. He has also, not unexpectedly, found an abnormally high family history of diabetes in this group.

Turning to minerals, Dr. Cott said that little is known at present about our requirements for the trace minerals, and that we know even less about all the complex interaction among various trace minerals, vitamins and other food elements. In children who show disorders of blood sugar regulation, he has found disturbance of histamine levels and trace minerals as well. In 26 of 30 children, he found lower than normal levels of several minerals in analyzing hair for mineral content. Lead was present in every sample tested.

We have been told that the trace mineral zinc is present in ample quantity in our food supply. Today there is evidence that this may not be so. Zinc is an important constituent in the body activity that goes on involving chromium, zinc and magnesium, as well as the hormone insulin, essential for regulating blood sugar levels. An excess of other minerals which cannot be avoided may interfere with the body's use of the essential ones. You can readily see how complicated this matter is and how far we can stray from natural, healthful conditions when we begin to tamper with food in the manufacturing and processing operations.

And what of the soil in which the food is grown? Dr. Cott cheerfully takes on the entire chemical and agricultural empire near the end of his article when he says: "Plants grown on a well fertilized soil should contain all the trace elements vital to life. However, the soils of all lands are not adequate, for many of them have been cultivated for a century with fertilizers containing only nitrate, phosphate, potash, calcium and magnesium. These fertilizers grow plants with inadequate levels of trace minerals.

"The use of organic fertilizers or compost provides more of the trace elements," he continued. "The sandy soil of Florida lacks many of the trace elements necessary to grow an abundant citrus crop. At present, zinc, manganese, cobalt, molybdenum, iron and copper salts are all added to the citrus groves." Organic gardening and farming, we might add, would probably solve these problems of trace mineral lack.

And what of the heavy metals that are polluting more and more of the earth? Dr. Cott said that research in England seems to show extremely high levels of lead in the blood of city children. He quotes one expert who says that no other toxic pollutant has accumulated in man to average levels so close to the threshold for overt clinical poisoning. Then he tells of another researcher who found that a group of mentally retarded children had distinctly more lead in their blood than a group of normal children. In fact, he said, "nearly half the retarded children had higher blood levels of lead than the maximum level in the other group."

Lead is in the air wherever heavy traffic goes using leaded gasoline. Almost nothing has been done to get the lead out of gasoline, although lots of speeches and promises have been made. We also get lead in food and water. City children in poor districts who eat flakes of paint from the walls are threatened with lead poisoning if the paint is lead-based. It is, therefore, encouraging to read in *The New York Times* for March 11, 1972 that the Food and Drug Administration has banned all except trace amounts of lead in paint for interior use by the end of 1973 "to minimize the health hazard to future generations."

Summing up his work and the work of others in treating mentally disturbed children, those who cannot speak, cannot learn, cannot control their hyperactivity, Dr. Cott explained, "Investigation of this treatment modality by controlled studies should be given the highest priority, for we are dealing with a patient population of 20 million children."

Dr. Abram Hoffer, whom we mentioned earlier, has had remarkable results with niacin and vitamin C in treating problem children. Writing in *Schizophrenia* in 1971, Dr. Hoffer reported that he used three to 12 grams of niacin and three grams of vitamin C daily. He also emphasized good nutrition. "Any psychiatrist who begins with a cohort of 100 acute schizophrenics and follows the orthomolecular approach for a sufficient length of time, say three years, will find that 90% of his patients are well, the rest improved, none will be worse."

The outcome of a nutritional survey of over 600 children from New York City's lower East Side, released in 1968, indicated that not all American children are well nourished. Poor diets, low vitamin levels and below average size and weight were found in certain groups of children in an analysis by New Jersey College of Medicine and Dentistry physicians, a New York physician and a statistician. In one group of Puerto Rican children, low levels of vitamin C, niacin and vitamin B12 were found. These same children had low reading levels, a finding which points to the need for good nutrition in order to perform well in school. This was in contrast with a group of Chinese children who showed very high reading scores. These youngsters were on good diets and had high levels of thiamine and pyridoxine. In the Chinese group, 30% took supplementary vitamins.

A striking feature of another group of children was very low riboflavin levels. "The importance of riboflavin deficiency as a general nutritional problem has been emphasized," the investigators noted. These children were also low in all B vitamins except folic acid and thiamine, as well as vitamin C.

In one group, low levels of vitamin B2, B6 and B12 were discovered. Most of these children came from families in which the mother was the main wage earner. "The mother's absence during the day may explain the frequent finding of a poor dietary history," the report added. "Maternal neglect or rejection has been shown to be correlated with decreased height, weight and bone maturation."

Add to this report the following note from the Metropolitan Life Insurance Company: In 1966, about 3,629,000 babies were born in the United States and about 84,800 died in their first year of life. These figures translate into a rate of 23.4 infant deaths per 1,000 live births, a figure that suggests plenty of room for improvement. Comparing these figures with those of other countries, the Metropolitan statisticians found that we are 15th among all nations in figures on infant mortality. All the following countries lose fewer babies each year than we do: Scotland, France, Israel, Japan, Czechoslovakia, England and Wales, Switzerland, Australia, Denmark, New Zealand, Finland, Norway, Netherlands and Sweden.

Could not these figures be the outcome of conditions of wretchedly poor nutrition among whole groups of people in our country? These reports are only two in a long series of surveys over the years, several of which we have mentioned in this book, all of which have shown that considerable numbers of our young people are sadly deficient in essential nutrients. In the case of children studied in New York, their plight is doubly alarming. Surrounded by poverty, filth, poor housing, noise, pollution, many of these children are destined to become the patients we have been discussing. No one knows how much of the reason for this may be simple lack of vitamins, minerals and protein in their diets.

One added statistic: a headline in *The New York Times* for November 3, 1967 states, "19 Million Children Termed Poverty-Stricken in U.S." This report, issued by the Citizens Committee for Children of New York, asserted that there is an urgent need for some form of family or children's allowance program to combat this wide area of poverty. We suspect that this sad news can be repeated in all of the major metropolitan areas of the nation.

From time to time we hear reports of various investigations by resourceful scientists of the possible relationship between crime and poor nutrition. Undoubtedly, it is difficult to sort out all the many environmental elements that enter into the personality of any one person. Someone who commits a serious crime is no exception. Probably both heredity and home, school and community environment are responsible for the kind of individual who is driven to commit a murder, an armed robbery, a rape.

Now we have evidence from an Egyptian physician that lack of niacin may have a great deal to do with the personality of the criminal. You will remember that Dr. Glen Green suggested this same theory earlier in this chapter. According to *Schizophrenia,* Dr. El Kholy said he had studied crime and pellagra from 1941 to 1948. Once again, Dr. Kholy confirmed that the symptoms of pellagra can easily be mistaken for a schizophrenic personality. He examined 1,150 people who had been accused of serious crimes, and he found that 206 or 18% had pellagra. Their crimes included murder, threats to kill, attempted murder, serious assault, kidnap, arson, rape, etc. Over one-third of all who were later declared to be insane murderers were found to have pellagra.

Said the article: "Had pellagra been prevented, there would have been a major decrease in crimes of violence. By analogy, if elimination of pellagra reduces crimes of violence, how much more will eradication of schizophrenia achieve? It is suggested, therefore, that perhaps the addition of vitamin B3 to our food in doses of one gram per day or more will do for schizophrenia what the fortification of flour with much smaller doses of nicotinamide (niacin) has done for pellagra."

Additional information on the use of vitamin therapy in dealing with schizophrenia can be obtained from the Huxley Institute for Biosocial Research, 56 W. 45th St., Suite 805, New York City 10036.

CHAPTER 6

Alcoholism and The B Complex

WHAT IS ALCOHOLISM? According to the American Medical Association, it is a disease, like cancer or diabetes. Alcohol is a mind-altering drug, which has the qualities of inducing tolerance and withdrawal symptoms—two qualities which are associated with physiological dependence or addiction. This happens after a varying, but usually long preliminary period of heavy social drinking. We don't yet know why one out of every 15 adult U. S. drinkers ends up as an alcoholic. Why don't the other 14?

Unfortunately, nobody knows the answer to this basic question, and surprisingly little is being done to find out, considering the prevalence of the disease. There are more than 6½ million

Americans suffering from alcoholism, according to Dr. Roger O. Egeberg of the Department of Health, Education and Welfare. He has described alcoholism as the nation's number one neglected health problem. Statistics show that the average untreated alcoholic's life-span is shortened by 12 years, yet most cases of alcoholism in the United States fail to get adequate and nutritional attention. Early symptoms often go unrecognized because U. S. physicians are not adequately trained to detect them. Alcoholism still suffers from the effects of social and moral prejudices which retard its recognition as an illness and, therefore, discourage urgently needed professional treatment.

If your answer is "yes" to any of the following key questions, prepared by the National Council on Alcoholism, you have some of the symptoms that *may* indicate incipient alcoholism:

1. Difficult to get along with when drinking.
2. Drinks "because he is depressed."
3. Drinks "to calm his nerves."
4. Drinks until he is "dead drunk" at times.
5. Can't remember parts of some episodes.
6. Hides liquor.
7. Lies about his drinking.
8. Neglects to eat when he is drinking.

If you even *suspect* that you are slowly drifting into alcoholism, you should seek expert advice right away. There may be a local Alcoholics

Anonymous chapter close to your home. If you wish, you may contact the National Council on Alcoholism, 2 Park Ave., New York City. Even if you are lucky enough not to have an alcohol problem yourself, you can help others who do, with a check to the just-named Council.

The precise roles of the physical disposition and psychological factors and the combination of psychology, predisposition and cultural availability of alcohol in the genesis of alcoholism are not known. It is not impossible that a lab test for susceptibility to alcoholism could be found. Research on these many variables in alcoholism is much needed and is a goal of the NCA.

Chemical aspects of alcoholism provide an exciting subject for future study. Fortunately, however, effective and tested methods of rehabilitation are already available, and have proven highly successful in literally hundreds of thousands of cases. The key to rehabilitation for today's alcoholic rests largely in the hands of his fellow citizens. It is *they* who must realize how impossible it is for an alcoholic to fight against his addiction without competent professional help. They must see to it that he gets such help as easily as possible.

Like many other diseases that get worse by degrees, alcoholism is difficult to spot but easiest to treat in its early stages. The time that separates heavy drinking from alcoholism is a thin one. Yet the physician, who should be an expert in the detection of all disease, is often poorly equipped by his early training to detect the incipient signs.

What kind of people are alcoholics? Many of them are women. Few alcoholics are the "Skid Row Bum" variety, less than 5%. A high proportion of alcoholics are well-off in a financial way, and many hold high-paying jobs, which they are gradually forced to neglect as their disease gets worse, unless they are among the lucky few who now receive treatment. Many are teen-agers. And who hasn't heard about the middle-class, bored housewife who begins to hit the bottle for no readily discernible reason?

Many alcoholics have a lot of "strength of character" by anybody's standards. Yet they become alcoholics. Why? Much work remains to be done to disclose the answer. Alcoholics have in common only the fact that their daily intake of the drug—alcohol—exceeds their body's ability to handle it effectively.

Those of us who drink socially—even if we are quite moderate drinkers—could be prone to the disease of alcoholism. For this reason, if for no other, we must all try to help establish a climate of public opinion which recognizes alcoholism for what it is—a disease—and to support the establishment of expanded research and treatment facilities.

These comments are from a news release from the National Council on Alcoholism. We think they are excellent as far as they go. Like practically all other statements by an official body, they end by saying that alcoholism is a disease and that a treatment of this disease must be found. Already many researchers have shown the cause and the treatment of alcoholism. Their research is virtually ignored by most of these official groups.

For quite some time alcoholism has been treated by diet—the same high protein, low-carbohydrate diet with frequent meals which keeps blood sugar levels on an even keel. Records of this successful treatment for alcoholism are available in a fine book, *Body, Mind and Sugar*, by E. M. Abrahamson and A. W. Pezet, in the previously mentioned *New Hope for Incurable Diseases*, by E. Cheraskin and W. Ringsdorf, and others.

In 1967, it was discovered that a New York physician cures alcoholics—even those who are in delirium tremens (DTs)—by making an opening in their stomachs and inserting a tube through which he feeds them a high protein liquid food, plus all the known vitamins and essential minerals.

Writing in the *Journal of the American Geriatrics Society* (September 1967), Dr. Frank S.

Butler noted that he must operate on his patients because they are so dependent on alcohol and so little accustomed to eating nourishing diets that they cannot feed themselves consistently with this preparation. But, as soon as the matter is taken out of their hands and they are literally forced to be well fed, whether they want to be or not, their health improves at once and they have no difficulty in changing their usual drinking habits.

Dr. Roger J. Williams and his co-workers at the University of Texas have made alcoholics out of mice by giving them inadequate diets and then making either alcohol or water available for drinking. This resulted in producing alcoholism in about the same proportion of mice as there are people afflicted with the disease. Dr. Williams interpreted this as meaning that individual mice, like individual human beings, have varying needs for nutrients. If these needs are satisfied by the individual's diet, he does not "take to alcohol," but can drink or not, as he wishes, without becoming addicted. Dr. Williams could also "cure" his alcoholic mice by giving them diets high enough in protein, vitamins and minerals to meet their individual nutritional needs.

On the other hand, if diet is not providing for these extra nutrients the individual desperately needs, he will try to quiet his quivering nerves and raise his sagging self-confidence by drinking alcohol to excess. The more he drinks, the more badly nourished be becomes, for alcohol contains nothing but calories, hence, nothing nourishing. The alcoholic, through no fault of his own, is thus led into a vicious cycle which finally results in his death—usually from malnutrition. For a more detailed discussion of the nutritional origins of alcoholism, we strongly recommend Dr. Williams' latest book, *Nutrition Against Disease*, published in 1971 by the Pitman Publishing Co., New York City. His other books, all containing valuable nutritional information, include: *You Are Extraordinary, Nutrition in a Nutshell, Alcoholism: The Nutritional Approach, Biochemical Individuality* and *Nutrition and Alcoholism*. The older books (except *Nutrition and Alcoholism*, which is no longer available) are probably in your local library; the newer ones are sold in most health food stores and book shops.

Said Dr. Butler: "Alcoholism can be controlled with a diet high in protein and rich in vitamins, especially the B vitamins. Since the alcoholic cannot be expected to accept a change in diet, he must be fed involuntarily." Thus, Dr. Williams proved successfully that alcoholism can be induced by a diet that does not meet individual needs and can be "cured" by a diet which does. Dr. Abrahamson showed that an excellent high-protein diet, taken at frequent intervals during the day, can provide enough of all nutrients to enable the alcoholic to climb back on the wagon permanently and stay there, as long as he adheres to the high-protein diet.

Dr. Butler, who at the time of the article was with Columbus Hospital in New York, further elaborates on his thesis by saying that the alcoholic is powerless to control his drinking, that he progresses to a debilitated condition by rejecting food, except for alcohol, so that symptoms increase, the liver is affected and, finally, there is malnutrition and vitamin deficiency, which result in "irreversible and inevitable end-results." He goes on to say that all the arguments in the fields of medicine, psychology and sociology have brought no solution.

"The physiology of the body demands essential nutrition in the form of carbohydrates, fats, proteins and vitamins. Any of these elements of diet if ingested to the exclusion of the others result in an unbalanced fuel intake . . . Alcohol is an easily absorbed, rapidly utilized source of energy in the form of calories only . . . Alcohol taken to excess satisfies the immediate energy requirement, but the associated malnutrition and avitaminosis (a deficiency in vitamins) are manifested by fatty degeneration of the functioning organs of the body," Dr. Butler said.

Dr. Butler describes the treatment of a patient

who had been a hopeless alcoholic for six years. He had not worked for three years and was admitted to the hospital in a state of acute DTs with an accumulation of fluid in his lungs. He was taken to the operating room, a tube was inserted in his stomach, and he was fed the scientifically calculated liquid food that is predigested and placed directly into the patient's stomach. The tube is plugged on the outside and the patient is given the liquid diet to take home if he wishes, or he can use it for only some meals by inserting it into the tube, after he has once again established nutritious eating habits. Within 48 hours this particular patient was walking around, needing nothing more than the prescribed feedings. After three months he had gained 30 pounds and was working steadily.

In his article, Dr. Butler gives two other examples of this treatment and states that it is feasible for use in all other cases. The nutritional deficiency will be corrected and the nutritional complications of chronic alcoholism will be avoided.

Swedish physicians have found that a dose of vitamins taken before drinking alcoholic beverages will help the drinker to feel less drunk. Dr. Leonard Goldberg used policemen in his test. Eight of them received shots in the arm of large doses of the B vitamins. Eight others were injected with fluid that contained nothing of any value. Then all of them were given large amounts of alcohol. Those who had received the vitamin B reported less feelings of intoxication and, in tests of perception and reaction, they tested higher than the other policemen who had received the placebo. Why not take a whopping dose of the B vitamins before you go to the next cocktail party and see what your own reactions are?

Muscle damage in chronic alcoholics may result from independent actions of the alcohol itself and not simply from a nutritional deficiency in the alcoholic, according to *Science* for January 21, 1972, and discussed in a press release from the National Institutes of Health, which helped to fund the study. Drs. Sun K. Song and Emanuel Rubin of the Department of Pathology, Mount Sinai School of Medicine, New York, reported increased serum enzyme activity (serum creatine phosphokinase) and ultrastructural changes in skeletal muscles of three men who consumed excessive amounts of alcohol for 28 days while maintaining an otherwise balanced diet. Muscle damage (myopathy) afflicts alcoholic humans in two forms, the NIH reported. Acute alcoholic myopathy is characterized by muscle pain, tenderness and edema (swelling). Chronic alcoholic myopathy is a progressive state of weakness: muscle cells may die or wash away; tissues may become inflamed; certain cell components may be destroyed.

"For about 15 years, physicians have recognized an association between muscle damage and continuous consumption of alcohol," the National Institutes of Health stated. "However, they have been unable to identify the exact cause of myopathy as either a manifestation of the toxic quality of the alcohol itself or the result of the dietary deficiencies, malnutrition and other conditions which often accompany alcoholism. Drugs have also induced myopathy, clinically and experimentally.

"In previous studies of the effects of alcohol consumption on muscles, scientists have confined their observation to chronic alcoholics for whom reliable histories of dietary habits, drug ingestion and amount of alcohol consumed are difficult to obtain. In the present study, however, the grantees examined the effects of ethanol (common alcohol) in humans under controlled conditions," the NIH said.

It is interesting to note that one New York City manufacturer claims to have a cure for hangover, that depressing combination of upset stomach, headache, nausea, dizziness, etc., that follows excessive drinking. The ingredients for the tablets include "two pain relievers for headache, three antacids for upset stomach, two B vitamins that alcohol removes from the body, oil of peppermint for gas and a stimulant to pick you up and combat depression," the company stated.

While on the subject of hangover, perhaps we should mention that another New York manufacturer insists that activated charcoal in capsule or tablet form may spell the end to morning-after hangover. This was reported in the September 9, 1971 issue of the *Journal of Southwestern Medicine*.

At "The Crisis in Health Care for the Aging" conference, sponsored by The Huxley Institute for Biosocial Research on March 6, 1972 at the Hilton Hotel in New York, Dr. Roger J. Williams had some significant remarks to make about nutrition and alcoholism.

"There are two energy-yielding chemicals commonly consumed for which self-selection often fails to work advantageously. One is sugar. The other is alcohol," Dr. Williams said.

"Children who are raised on soft drinks and given a choice will choose more of the same in preference to nourishing foods. Adults who commonly consume alcoholic beverages regularly and copiously for long periods of time not infrequently reach the point where they lose interest in nourishing food and have, on the contrary, a prevailing interest in consuming alcoholic beverages," he added.

"In each case, the appetite controlling mechanism in the brain goes awry. In children, excess sugar consumption leads to general malnutrition," Dr. Williams continued. "In adults, consuming too much alcohol can lead not only to general malnutrition but also to severe damage of the brain. Brains of alcoholics are so badly damaged that their cadavers are unfit for brain dissection by medical students.

"Alcoholism is a terrific health hazard and elderly people are highly susceptible, particularly if they have had extended drinking experience," Dr. Williams said. He noted that it often takes several years of heavy drinking before a person becomes an alcoholic. The effect is also cumulative and elderly people who are affluent and have a long history of alcoholism or alcohol consumption are particularly vulnerable, he said.

"It has long been my opinion that good nutrition is a key to the prevention of alcoholism and that biochemical individuality plays a tremendous role in that some individuals have unusual needs which may make them highly vulnerable. If, however, nutritional education can be advanced to the point where the public will concentrate on wholesome food, alcoholism will be abolished," the distinguished Texas scientist said.

Dr. Williams said that the simplest insurance against alcoholism is good, wholesome food. This not only furnishes the necessary energy —that is the calories required—but also the wherewithal to build and maintain healthy cells.

"A simple nutritional rule, if followed, would prevent alcoholism from ever developing. It is this—that no more than 10% of the calories one consumes day by day be naked or empty calories," Dr. Williams said. "If 90% of the calories one consumes are in the form of wholesome food, malnutrition will not become a part of life; individuals will never pass through a period of preparation for drinking, which is the *sine qua non* or prerequisite of becoming an alcoholic."

Another speaker at the same seminar was Dr. George Christakis, Professor of Community Medicine (Nutrition), Mount Sinai School of Medicine in New York. His address concerned the many problems of the aging, including inadequate income, decreased mobility (in terms of disability, lack of motivation, too many stairs or other impediments), and, a No. 1 problem in many neighborhoods—crime in the streets. He noted that it is "impossible to buy a nutritious diet for the elderly with some of the welfare benefits currently received."

"Now, getting more specifically to alcohol, ethanol (another name for alcohol) contains seven calories a gram and thus is more related to the caloric content of fat, rather than carbohydrate," Dr. Christakis said. "Inasmuch as good survivorship and leanness are related, the contribution of alcohol to the problem of obesity which, in turn, is related to longevity, may be a real one. It is more likely that the social alcoholic who eats adequately as well as drinks will become obese rather than the severe alcoholic who drinks but does not eat adequately. Certainly the tremendous advertising campaign to promote the drinking of alcohol is made to the old as well as the young."

The absorption of alcohol into the blood stream is directly from the stomach, and there is no impaired deficiency with aging, Dr. Christakis said. "It is postulated, however, that aging may modify and complicate alcoholism in two ways. First, by inducing decreased speech, spacial and motor coordination secondary to cerebral arteriosclerosis (hardening of the arteries) with enhancement of the effect of alcohol on the central nervous system due to possibly decreased neural (nerve) threshold responses.

"Second, since vitamins are components of co-enzymes involved in the efficient oxidation of alcohol, absolute or relative deficiencies of these micro-nutrients may delay degradation of alcohol and heighten or prolong its pharmacologic response. Experimental thiamine deficiencies in animals," Dr. Christakis then continued, "do not appear to alter the rate of alcohol metabolism. However, the diuretic (secretion through the urine) effect of alcohol may incite vitamin losses and thus compromise stores (of the vitamins in the body)."

Dr. Christakis said that, if there is a fatty liver present in the early stages of alcoholism, the presence of the alcohol blocks the lipo-proteins —not from forming but from leaving the liver. This might be the first stage to the fatty liver and to the cirrhosis that follows. Dr. Christakis added that cirrhosis can usually be reversed simply by stopping the alcohol.

"Incidentally, there is much macrocytic anemia associated with alcoholism in the elderly, and Herbert and his co-workers have found that there seems to be a block even when they give folic acid," Dr. Christakis said.

Alcohol seems to block the proper action of bone marrow in manufacturing healthy blood cells. Even 100 milligrams of folic acid a day cannot correct the situation unless the alcohol is stopped.

Low potassium and magnesium have also been found in elderly alcoholics, the New York researcher said. He added that this may be related to the DTs of alcoholism in the elderly as well as the middle-aged.

He noted that, since there is cellular loss, particularly in the aging, there must be adequate nutrition, particularly to replace the lack of critical amino acids and those vitamins involved in protein synthesis—namely, folic acid and vitamin B12; and, unless you have good nutrition, this would mitigate against optimal cellular replacement.

"Nutritional factors would seem to be all the more important since, in animal experiments, it has been shown that protein synthesis does not decrease with age, as measured by cyclical protein deprivation and refeeding," Dr. Christakis said.

Dr. Chauncey D. Leake had a word of warning for everyone, regardless of age. "You should never insult your stomach by putting into it anything stronger than 20% alcohol. That is about the limit of the concentration of the fortified wines," he said.

"The alcohol in wines or beers can be rapidly absorbed. It goes through the body quickly and has all kinds of effects, including dilation of blood vessels, taking a load off the heart," Dr. Leake said.

Dr. Leake did not object to a moderate and judicious use of wines and beers among nonalcoholic oldsters. "It has been found in many institutions that the (confinement) that has been complained of can be alleviated to a considerable extent by a social hour in which wine is deliberately served. This has worked superbly at Framingham, for example. We do it all over California," Dr. Leake continued.

Later, during a question-and-answer period, someone asked Dr. Leake how much alcohol you could consume before becoming an alcoholic, if you are eating a well-balanced diet.

"That would depend on your individual enzyme systems, but I would say that you had better not consume very much," he said. "Moderation is certainly the point. When I advocated the use of wines and beers as an adjunct to gracious living and pleasant eating, I meant to imply, of course, that they are under a certain degree of social control and regulation. Nothing to excess.

"This is an ancient idea, of course," Dr. Leake added. "Moderation in everything. And, if we could live up to what the Greeks suggested to us 2,500 years ago, I think we would all be better."

Dr. Roger J. Williams added another interesting observation about alcoholism. "In my rather long clinical psychiatric experience, I have come to the conclusion that there is a qualitative difference between alcoholism occurring in people before age 35 and alcoholism occurring in the old-age category, say 55 or 60 and beyond.

"This is because, in most of the instances where I have treated what looked like a real alcoholism in an older person, it was much more readily reversible and even curable in the sense that the person could go back to social drinking. This is almost impossible with the young alcoholic.

"The reason for this is that, in the older person, alcoholism is often based on depression," Dr. Williams said. "He is depressed and uses alcohol as his tranquilizer. In the younger person, depression follows alcoholism. In other words, it is a product of alcoholism."

CHAPTER 7

Pyridoxine

VITAMIN B6—or pyridoxine—has long been in the forefront of the health-seekers' drive against ill-health. Over the past 15 years or so, medical and scientific literature has produced a wealth of information about the essential nature of this B vitamin. But, for the most part, its importance has been overlooked by the official spokesmen on nutrition. "Everyone gets enough of it in the average diet," they are apt to say.

It was not until 1968 that the official pace-setters for nutrition—the National Academy of Sciences-National Research Council—decided that pyridoxine is, indeed, essential for human welfare and must be included in their official lists of Recommended Dietary Allowances of vitamins and minerals.

In November, 1968, a symposium of the New York Academy of Sciences was devoted entirely to this vitamin and its place in human nutrition. Prominent among the speakers was Dr. David Coursin of a Lancaster, Pennsylvania hospital, who has done a great deal of work on the effects of pyridoxine deficiency in newborn children. During the first weeks of life, he told the symposium, a deficiency in this nutrient affects brain development with symptoms including excessive irritability, defective behavior and convulsive seizures. Brain-wave patterns are abnormal and tests reveal that the kidneys are excreting abnormal amounts of certain proteins. How can this deficiency be corrected? By giving pyridoxine in enormous doses—100 milligrams at a time. (The official daily recommendation for a baby is 0.2 milligram per day). All symptoms disappear within minutes after these large doses of the vitamin are given.

Another specialist, Dr. Jack A. Klieger and his colleagues at a Milwaukee hospital, suggested that lack of pyridoxine may be responsible for toxemia of pregnancy, a disorder that kills some 30,000 infants and hundreds of mothers every year. It is possible, he said, that inability to use the vitamin properly may be the cause, along with lack of large enough amounts of the B vitamin.

Dr. Raymond E. Brown of the University of

Wisconsin spoke on the relationship between female hormones and pyridoxine. When a woman is pregnant, or when she takes hormone-rich contraceptive pills (which create a false pregnancy in her body), the amount of this female hormone, estrogen, rises. Testing pregnant women and women taking The Pill, Dr. Brown found them to be deficient in vitamin B6. They, too, were excreting abnormal amounts of proteins in their urine, until large doses of pyridoxine restored all these functions to normal.

Said Dr. Brown: "It probably would be sensible for pregnant women to take vitamin B6, though we're not in a position to say a deficiency is a real hazard. The implication of our findings is unclear."

There is nothing unclear about another extremely important function of pyridoxine—helping to prevent bladder cancer. In the absence of this vitamin, one of the proteins in food breaks down into excessive amounts of certain substances which then pass into the bladder for excretion. These products resemble chemicals which are known to cause cancer. Therefore, it seems clear that deficiency of pyridoxine may be responsible for causing bladder cancer in susceptible persons.

A number of years ago, a commercial baby formula caused convulsions in newborn children taking it, which resulted in mental deficiency in some of these babies. Mystified physicians who reported the cases and found they were all related to this one food discovered eventually that the way the formula was processed destroyed all of the pyridoxine. They injected the vitamin into the children who were ill and the convulsions stopped immediately, although in some cases permanent brain damage remained.

The doctors and scientists who studied these cases could not understand why some children who ate the faulty formula were affected while others were not. They finally came to the only possible conclusion—that some individuals need more of this important vitamin than others. Those whose needs were less somehow managed to get along on whatever pyridoxine remained in their tissues after birth, while the affected children could not survive healthfully for even a few days without the B vitamin.

The formula was withdrawn from the market and supposedly this particular threat to newborn babies is over. But an article in the February 7, 1965 issue of the *Journal of the American Medical Association* seems to prove otherwise. A Utah physician reported in this article on two babies who had convulsions several hours after birth. One of them died. The other was given massive doses of sedatives and other drugs and became rapidly worse. An injection of 100 milligrams of pyridoxine quieted the convulsions and brought the infant back to normal. But several times after this, the child required larger doses of the B vitamin and finally she was put on a daily dose. Said the author, "Daily maintenance therapy of four to 10 milligrams, administered orally, is necessary to maintain the child symptom free." No one knew how long the child would have to take the vitamin. One such child, eight years old, still needed the vitamin to prevent convulsions.

The Utah physician reported that, in several families, more than one child had been so affected. This seems to indicate that the need for large amounts of pyridoxine is inherited. If the obstetrician knows about cases like this, he will give the child vitamin B6 immediately and thus prevent permanent damage. If he does not, the convulsions may progress to fatality or may so damage the child's brain that recovery is impossible. The article recommends that all infants with convulsions be given an immediate large dose of pyridoxine. So every infant who is thus afflicted at birth should have the benefit of this injection, in case pyridoxine deficiency is responsible.

In the *New England Journal of Medicine*, July 17, 1969, a Yale University professor discusses two B vitamins in relation to differing needs for them and theorizes on what this may mean for nutrition study and good health. Dr.

Leon E. Rosenberg tells us that just not getting enough of one or several vitamins can result in certain symptoms which can be alleviated by giving the individual food that contains these vitamins. But a need for larger amounts than average of a vitamin is quite a different thing. This need is something that we must inherit. Our parents may suffer from the same trouble, or, in the complicated maze of genetic happenings, one parent may bequeath a child this heritage. In some cases, perhaps a mother may be only a "carrier" of the genetic fault, passing it along to her sons, although she does not suffer from it.

How could such a genetic fault be related to vitamins? Very easily. Vitamins work with amino acids to change them into substances needed to nourish cells. If, because of an inherited fault, something goes awry with the way one's body uses an amino acid, the vitamin that is involved in some specific activity with the amino acid may be required in enormous doses by such an individual. Just the amount available in food does not suffice. And the condition is not called vitamin deficiency; it's called vitamin dependency.

Pyridoxine was one of the vitamins that Dr. Rosenberg discussed. He reviewed the story of the infants with convulsions, which we have just related, and reported that adults suffering from such a deficiency do not have convulsions, but they have "vague" symptoms of weakness, fatigue and lack of appetite, along with a kind of anemia that does not respond to iron medication or other drugs which cure other kinds of anemia. It does respond to administration of pyridoxine.

Then Dr. Rosenberg says that there are five known inherited disorders in which vitamin B6 is involved—that is, five conditions in which the vitamin is "dependent". These conditions are named after some of the biological and chemical events that take place in the afflicted person: pyridoxine-responsive anemia, cystathioninuria, xanthurenic acidura, homocystinuria and infantile convulsions. In every case, the only possible treatment is enormous amounts of the vitamin.

The other vitamin that Dr. Rosenberg discussed was vitamin B12. He noted that some of the same inherited differences as with pyridoxine are apparent. Vitamin B12 is manufactured almost exclusively by bacteria in soil, in water and in the digestive organs of animals, including man. We need so little of this vitamin that it is supposedly easy to get enough in any diet that includes animal protein. Vegetarians who eat no animal food can develop a vitamin B12 deficiency.

But there is a certain something called "intrinsic factor" which exists in the normal digestive tract which must be present for this vitamin to be absorbed. If you lack this, all the vitamin B12 in your daily meals may do you no good and you may develop a case of pernicious anemia which, untreated, can be a fatal disease. The lack of this absorbing factor is an inherited defect. There are other circumstances, too—man-made ones—which may interfere with absorption of this essential vitamin: operations for instance, where parts of the digestive tract have been removed.

Dr. Rosenberg believes that babies may have an inherited need for enormous amounts of vitamin B12, even though their symptoms may not indicate pernicious anemia. Such children get along fine while they are taking massive doses of the vitamin, and return to their diseased state if the vitamin is withdrawn. The scientist discusses all the extremely complex mechanisms which may be involved in the way the body uses or misuses this vitamin, depending solely on what one's inheritance is.

Added Dr. Rosenberg: "The events of the last decade presage increasing recognition of new genetic disorders that demonstrate vitamin dependency." When he was asked later what other vitamins might be involved in similar genetic tangles, he replied: "There are really as many possibilities as there are vitamins . . . I think it is very likely that thiamine, riboflavin, biotin and other vitamins that function as coenzymes will be shown to be effective in modifying specific inborn errors. . . We need much more information on this point."

A lack of pyridoxine has been found to be related to a very serious kind of anemia. According to two researchers, writing in *Blood*, May, 1964, animals completely deprived of vitamin B6 for about a year developed the anemia, which disappeared when the B vitamin was restored to their diets.

The Archives of Dermatology reported a case of *herpes gestationis* (inflammation of the legs during the fourth week of pregnancy), which did not respond to medication. There was a dramatic remission while the patient was on a high dosage of pyridoxine, which was continued up until the twenty-fifth week of pregnancy when it was no longer needed. The dosage was 10 milligrams a day.

A West German physician reported in *Medical World News* for June 25, 1965 that unexplained cerebral spasms or noticeable restlessness and nervousness in early infancy may be due to pyridoxine deficiency. He described one child which showed these symptoms within one hour after birth. He cautions that such children must be given up to 60 milligrams daily over long periods of time to prevent retarded development.

Little is known how the 50-odd nutrients needed by man affect one another's requirements, according to an army doctor at Fitzsimmons General Hospital in Denver, Colorado. So he did some research on how vitamin C, pyridoxine and protein react with one another. He found, according to *Science News* for July 3, 1971, that, in people who are getting too little pyridoxine, blood levels of vitamin C dropped. When he added the B vitamin to their diets, the vitamin C in their blood rose again. Doing similar tests with protein, he found that the more protein volunteers were getting in their diets, the more pyridoxine they needed. The pyridoxine is needed to help the body handle the protein.

Writing in *Nutrition Reviews*, Dr. M. K. Horwitt said that more than 90% of all patients with mental disorders suffer from some metabolic problem. That is, some problem having to do with the way the body uses food. The brain uses 25% of all oxygen taken into the body, so it requires a massive blood supply of its own. Therefore, it is not surprising that the brain should be affected by nutrients, or lack of them, in the bloodstream. People lacking pyridoxine show definite aberrations in the brain-wave patterns, he stated.

In another issue of *Nutrition Reviews*, it was reported that experiments on rats showed that the pituitary contains far more pyridoxine than other glands. When a diet deficient in this B vitamin is eaten for several weeks, the pyridoxine content of the master gland falls to less than 2% of its normal level. It is believed that the pituitary gland controls the functions of all other body glands, so its well-being is essential. It is known to be important for both growth and reproduction, and the health of the nervous system.

Giving pyridoxine in cases of chronic gastritis associated with too little digestive juices has helped to improve the digestion of 18 patients, according to a Soviet physician. This was reported in *Medical World News* for October 8, 1965. Dr. M. S. Lamanskaya tested the vitamin in 30 patients and got improvement in 18. Some of these had too little hydrochloric acid in the digestive tract; some had the normal amount and some had too much. The doctor reports that this B vitamin greatly increases the digestion of protein, so she suggested that it should not be given to people with stomach ulcers, because she feels it might make the condition worse.

In *Medical Tribune* for December 8, 1971, a biochemist from the University of Pittsburgh, speaking at a symposium on Nutrition and the Future of Man, said that two B vitamins are essential for the production and transportation in the human body of antibodies—those materials which protect us from infections. The two vitamins are pyridoxine and pantothenic acid. In any individual who does not have enough of these vitamins in his body, the production of antibodies will be decreased. They will not circulate in the blood to accomplish their biological purpose, which is to destroy harmful bacteria. In addition, lack of pyridoxine tends to make one sensitive to various allergy-producing substances. When animals lack pyridoxine, their bodies are inefficient in manufacturing protein and nucleic acids, both of which are essential to life. When animals lack pantothenic acid, there seems to be a deficiency in the way the body transports proteins from where they are created inside cells to the outside where they are needed.

A Swedish journal, *Acta Societatis Medicorum Upsaliensis*, Volume 72, 1-2, 1967, reports a relationship between pyridoxine and the thyroid gland. Individuals who are suffering from a condition of hyperthyroidism appear to need more pyridoxine than normal people. The result is that there is a derangement of the way the body uses pyridoxine when the thyroid gland is disordered. The thyroid gland is located in the neck and is intimately concerned in a great many things that go on inside us. Its hormone, thyroxin, circulating to various parts of the body, helps to control growth and intelligence. It has a great influcnce on body weight and the rate at which we use or metabolize our food. An unhealthy thyroid gland also means disorders of the skin, the hair and the bone structure.

We know also that the mineral, iodine, is important for thyroid health, since it is used in making thyroxin. Now it appears that when the thyroid gland is overactive, the way the body uses pyridoxine is badly disordered. This could result in disordering all those functions which the B vitamin performs in the body.

In *Nutrition Reviews* for April 1967, we are told that pyridoxine may have something to do with preventing hardening of the arteries and heart troubles. When the vitamin is destroyed purposely in experiments, the amount of cholesterol in the blood rises sharply. It seems possible, from this, that getting enough of the B vitamin would help to prevent raised cholesterol levels of the blood, with their attendant dangers of heart attacks and strokes. The article stated that patients with hardening of the arteries were found to have very low levels of pyridoxine in their blood.

What could be the reason? The author of the *Nutrition Reviews* article suggests several. First, the people who have hardening of the arteries with low levels of pyridoxine may have excessively high requirements for vitamin B6. They may not have been getting enough in their diets before the disorder began. Or they may not be able to absorb sufficient amounts of pyridoxine at its normal concentration in the diet, and may need to have massive doses of it, even up to 100 milligrams a day.

In a similar vein, a New York Medical College researcher reports that he has found pyridoxine to be an anti-coagulant. Persons who have suffered blood clots causing heart attacks or strokes are often placed on anti-coagulant drugs, so that their blood will have a tendency to avoid clotting, thus avoiding another disastrous attack. But the physician in charge must watch the patient carefully, since too much of an anti-coagulant drug may give him a tendency to hemorrhage—which is just as dangerous as too-ready clotting.

According to Dr. Edward H. Mandel, who made this discovery, pyridoxine is a natural anti-coagulant in a concentration in the blood of 10 milligrams per cc. It is obvious that no purely natural food substance, taken in its natural form, will cause hemorrhaging. So it seems possible that pyridoxine may turn out to be the best anti-coagulant of them all, since there is no danger attached to its use. For the record, vitamin K is also necessary in promoting blood clotting and preventing hemorrhages. It is found most often in green vegetables, alfalfa leaves and fish meal.

"A number of diseases occur in man whose

principal therapeutic requirement is supplementation of the diet with pyridoxine," said a Canadian researcher writing in the *American Journal of Diseases of Children* for January 1967. Dr. Charles R. Scriver goes on to mention that people who do not properly absorb their food may be lacking in pyridoxine. This may either be because their digestive tracts do not absorb the vitamin or because it may not be transported correctly through cells and tissues. Or, he said, it may be destroyed by certain types of drugs. One which is known to destroy this B vitamin is isoniazid, which is used in treating tuberculosis. In some cases, pyridoxine may be lost through the kidneys. Certain disorders may inactivate the enzymes which make the vitamin available for the body. There may be an increased demand for the vitamin due to pregnancy or fever. Or the individual may just not be getting enough pyridoxine in his food.

This same medical journal, in April 1967, told of unborn infants who suffered from convulsions in the womb, apparently because of lack of the very large amounts of pyridoxine needed in their mother's diet. One child died after seven weeks, the second one died the day after birth, in a series of "lightning convulsions." The third one survived. The convulsions in the womb could be stopped by giving the pregnant woman large doses of pyridoxine. But these had to be continued for the child after it was born or it once again had convulsions. The authors suggest that a need for large amounts of vitamin B6 should be considered as a possible cause of abortions and stillbirths, especially in women who report convulsive movements of the unborn infant, or when convulsions occur soon after birth.

And in another issue of this journal, this time in October 1967, we learn that an important function of vitamins appears to be to protect us against harmful things to which we are exposed. Most often, the experts do not know why the vitamin acts as it does. They simply know that it exerts a kind of protective action in the face of some toxic substance.

Chloromycetin is a fairly new antibiotic, with a considerable potential for harm, if it is used in the wrong way, given in excessive doses or for prolonged periods of time to susceptible people. Hundreds of cases have been reported in medical literature in which the patients suffered anything from mild symptoms to death after taking this drug. Most commonly, the blood forming organs in the bone marrow were affected so that the patient suffered from a certain deadly kind of anemia.

The magazine reported on the case of a 12-year-old child with cystic fibrosis who was given chloromycetin and developed optic neuritis as a side effect. This is inflammation of the nerves of the eye, resulting in pain and difficulty in seeing. Each time she was given the antibiotic, the neuritis appeared. Then her doctors gave her very large doses of pyridoxine and vitamin B12, along with the antibiotic. There was no recurrence of the neuritis. And doses of the antibiotic given with the vitamins were considerably larger than the earlier doses had been. Presumably the child could continue to take the drug to combat the infection, and suffered no harm from it as long as the large doses of the B vitamins were given along with it.

The British journal, *Lancet*, for February 11, 1967 reported on a young girl who had a chronic condition in which a certain amino acid or protein was excreted in her urine. There were three such patients in two families. Giving pyridoxine in extremely large doses prevented the condition—which might have been inherited—and returned the child to good health. Related to the urine condition was a blood condition in which blood cells had a peculiar abnormal stickiness.

In the *New England Journal of Medicine* for April 7, 1966, it was reported that a young man with serious anemia was found to have excessively low levels of fats and cholesterol in his blood. One hundred milligrams of pyridoxine were given intramuscularly twice a day. The anemia was cured and the level of fatty substances in the blood became normal. But the patient had to continue to take the B vitamin every day. On three occasions when it was discontinued, the anemia returned within one or two months. The authors of the article believe that doctors treating such anemias should be on the lookout for other blood abnormalities that may accompany it. Interestingly enough, the young patient's parents were both alcoholic and he drank excessively.

Medical World News for January 15, 1965 reported that a Pennsylvania physician has found that children not getting enough pyridoxine "may become irritable, develop oversensitive hearing, and even suffer convulsions." Prompt detection and proper nutritional management is crucial, he said. The doctor gives daily doses of two to 10 milligrams of pyridoxine to such infants.

Parkinson's Disease is an affliction of the nerves which appears usually in middle-aged individuals. A drug (Levodopa) was recently developed which seems to improve greatly the Parkinson symptoms, but, at the same time, it produces very unpleasant side effects in the form of involuntary movements which the patient cannot control.

Doctors using this drug have known for some time that pyridoxine appears to be related in some mysterious way to the effects the drug has on the patient. In the June 28, 1971 issue of the *Journal of the American Medical Association,* two New York physicians tell of their experiences with one patient in whom they could control the Parkinson symptoms with Levodopa, but abnormal, uncontrollable movements then appeared. When they gave vitamin B6, these movements were controlled but the Parkinson symptoms appeared again.

By careful dosage, the doctors discovered that adding pyridoxine to the patient's medication was the equivalent of doubling the dose of Levodopa. They tried dosage with other patients and found that the same was true, except that the intensity of the effect of the B vitamin differed with different patients.

The doctors feel certain that this discovery will aid in future work with Parkinson patients. They can, by juggling dosages of the drug and the vitamin, produce improvement with few side effects, they hope. Hopefully, researchers will soon untangle the mystery of this difficult disorder. Is it possible that it may have its origin in lack of B vitamins?

Earlier in this chapter we discussed the pyridoxine research that was reported at a New York symposium in 1968. An earlier symposium, in July 1964, also brought together scientists from many countries who are working with vitamin B6. Here are some of the reports they gave:

1. Pyridoxine has an important role in pro-

cessing carbohydrate foods so that the body can use them effectively.

2. One-half of all the pyridoxine in the body is concentrated in the muscle. (Remember, the heart is a muscle).

3. There is a close relation between the amount of pyridoxine and fluctuations of blood sugar, indicating that deficiency in this vitamin may have something to do with both diabetes and low blood sugar.

4. An enzyme of which pyridoxine is a part has been found to be abundant in brain tissues. The amount of the vitamin is lower in old people. Could this lack be related to the mental health of the elderly?

5. Vitamin B6 is essential for the body to use protein efficiently. So one's intake of the vitamin should be related to one's intake of protein. The more protein you eat, the more pyridoxine you require.

6. Anyone deficient in pyridoxine cannot easily manufacture antibodies—those elements in the blood which help to protect against infections.

7. A University of California professor reported on experiments with monkeys which showed that animals deficient in pyridoxine developed hardening of the arteries very much like that which the human develops. In addition, deficient animals developed tooth decay—four

times that of animals whose diets were not deficient. Their tongues, gums and jaws also showed harmful effects. The livers of the deficient animals were enlarged, smooth and pale, while prolonged deficiency produced scarring in the livers.

8. A New York researcher reported that he had given pyridoxine lozenges containing 3 milligrams of the vitamin to teenagers, resulting in "significantly fewer" cavities in teeth. In 540 pregnant women, a lozenge containing 20 milligrams of vitamin B6 daily before and after the birth of their children results in "significantly" less incidence of tooth decay—even though all the women were drinking unfluoridated water.

9. Some kinds of anemia are cured with pyridoxine. Apparently the victims were having trouble using the iron in their food. A Cleveland scientist believes that they may suffer from an inherited "error of metabolism." In such cases, pyridoxine seems to effect a cure.

10. One researcher experimented with volunteers—young, healthy adults—who were put on a diet deficient in pyridoxine, although it was adequate in every other way. The young men soon began to suffer from abnormalities in the brain waves. One of them had an epileptic seizure during the seventh week of deficiency. This finding ties in with the incidents of the babies with convulsions that we have mentioned.

Pyridoxine is easily destroyed by sunlight and oxidation. This means that pyridoxine in milk stored in glass bottles has probably disappeared from the milk before we drink it. It also means that cutting or chopping foods long before they are eaten can result in total loss of this vitamin.

As we see from the chart on page 238, other foods which contain considerable amounts of vitamin B6 are whole grain cereals and flours; the organ meats like liver, heart and kidney; pork; veal; tuna and soybeans. Wheat germ contains more of this vitamin than any other food eaten in quantity; brewer's yeast contains about three times more than wheat germ. Blackstrap molasses is a close second, with almost twice the amount of pyridoxine found in wheat germ. Since white sugar contains no pyridoxine, it is easy to see that molasses is far superior in this one element, to say nothing of all its other vitamin and mineral riches.

Those of us who eat foods made from white flour are depriving ourselves of most of the pyridoxine that exists in the wheat berry. Wheat germ, that part of the wheat which is removed in refining and milling, contains up to 1,750 milligrams of vitamin B6 in 100 grams, which is an average serving. The bran of the wheat, which is also removed in milling, contains up to 1,570 milligrams. White flour, from which most of our bread is made, contains up to 600 milligrams per

100 grams. Of the wealth of vitamins and minerals that are removed in refining the wheat or other grain, only thiamine, riboflavin and niacin are replaced synthetically. However, one of the researchers at the 1964 symposium on pyridoxine believes that this vitamin, too, should be added to white flour.

The recommended dietary allowances for pyridoxine are: infants (0.2 to 0.4 milligrams daily); children (0.5 to 1.2 milligrams daily); males (1.4 to 2 milligrams daily); females (1.4 to 2 milligrams daily); pregnant women (2.5 milligrams daily); lactating women (2.5 milligrams daily).

CHAPTER 8

Pantothenic Acid

ACCORDING TO the Arthritis and Rheumatism Foundation in New York, arthritis is our most common chronic ailment and affects more than 12,000,000 Americans. In its most crippling form, it strikes hardest at the between 18- and 45-year-old age group. But, alarmingly, of the 12 million Americans who are afflicted, approximately 250,000 are children.

"Altogether," said the Foundation, "arthritis is responsible for an annual 115 million work days lost—a figure equivalent to 470,000 people out of work for a whole year. The experience of New York's Consolidated Edison Company is typical: among 1,000 employees, the company noted 168 full work days lost in one year because of arthritis.

Floyd B. Odlum, founder of the Atlas Corporation and board chairman of the Arthritis and Rheumatism Foundation, says the disease causes more disability and lost time from work than all accidents combined. It is second only to respiratory ailments as a cause of absenteeism, he said.

The Foundation has chronicled the percentage of arthritis sufferers in various occupational groups, as follows: factory workers (17%); craftsmen and foremen (13%); managers, store owners, company officials (10%); service workers (8.5%); clerical workers (7%); professional and technical workers (5%); sales workers (5%).

"Arthritis victims each lose an average of 15 work days out of the year; the total annual cost in lost wages is a startling $1.5 billion," the Foundation statement said.

"In addition, there is the annual $200 million lost income taxes from arthritics who can't work at all or who must switch to less demanding and usually lower-paying jobs," the Foundation continued. "Each year, some three million arthritics must change jobs or restrict their activities. In one year alone, taxpayers shelled out $194 million to support arthritics who were too crippled to work."

When you add together the medical expenses involved and the wages lost, you arrive at a $2 billion hole in the American economy each year, the Foundation said.

The Foundation further listed these warning signals that should send anyone to his doctor: 1) persistent pain and stiffness on arising, 2) pain or tenderness in at least one joint, 3) swelling in at least one joint, and 4) recurrence of these symptoms.

Concluded the Foundation: "At present, medical science knows no cure for arthritis . . . Research is turning up some promising leads; although the causes of rheumatoid arthritis remain unknown, scientists have found that certain conditions seem to bring on the disease—conditions such as shock, emotional or physical strain, fatigue, exposure to dampness and cold and chronic infections.

"Researchers are also working on the 'rheumatoid factor,' a giant protein molecule they have found in the blood of rheumatoid arthritis sufferers but not in normal blood. By supporting such research programs, and by helping their employees to escape the worst ravages of the disease, American industry can go far toward sewing up the $2 billion hole in the American pocket," the Foundation said.

While the search for a cure continues in the United States, three London scientists believe that arthritis is related to a lack of pantothenic acid in the blood. Discovered by Dr. Roger J. Williams, this B vitamin was named "pantothenic" from the Greek word meaning "derived from everywhere"—that is, present in many different forms. Dr. Williams has always felt that pantothenic acid should be taken in much larger amounts than the official recommendation.

He also believes that some people may have an inherited need for far larger amounts of this vitamin than other people. However, there does not seem to be any indication that people who suffer from arthritis eat diets deficient in this B vitamin. Rather, it seems, according to the experts, that the victims are deficient in the way their bodies use pantothenic acid.

Every vitamin, mineral and other food substance becomes involved in extremely complicated chemical changes as it is being digested and made into energy or cell structure in the body. During this process, the London researchers theorize, something is missing which the individual requires in order to use this B vitamin effectively.

They tested the blood of normal people and arthritics for its pantothenic acid content. In a healthy person they found that the level is about 107 micrograms in a given measure, whereas in arthritics it averages only about 68.7 micrograms. In fact they found, reports *Medical World News* for October 7, 1966, that any patient with less than 95 micrograms showed some symptoms of arthritis. And the lower the level of the B vitamin, the more severe the symptoms. A microgram, incidentally, is one-millionth of a gram.

In other tests, the English doctors found that several other substances which are closely involved with pantothenic acid in digestion were also at abnormal levels in arthritics. They injected into their patients these substances that were missing, and they gave daily injections of pantothenic acid for a month. There were no results. No improvement.

But the doctors were not so easily discouraged. They were sure some other substance must be missing, too. "We had one clue as to what this might be," said one of the scientists. "The richest natural source of pantothenic acid is royal jelly, the larval food of the queen bee." Royal jelly is also the richest source of another substance with the tongue-twisting name of 10-hydroxy-delta 2-decenoic acid.

The physicians injected pantothenic acid along with royal jelly into 20 of their rheumatoid arthritis patients. In 14 there was improvement in their symptoms. They were able to move more easily and other symptoms characteristic of the disease disappeared, so long as the patients continued to take the injections. Later, the doctors found a cheaper substitute for the very expensive and rare substance in royal jelly. And they found they could get results by giving this substance, along with pantothenic acid, by mouth rather than by injection.

Working with osteoarthritic patients, the London researchers added a substance called cysteine to the pantothenic acid and got excellent results with these patients. How much did they give? They had no guidelines to go by. So they experimented until they found the dosage that produced results.

Sometimes the results were slow in coming. There seems to be no improvement for the first four to eight weeks. But, said one of the doctors, "Just when the patient is deciding that the cure is no good, the symptoms disappear overnight." The treatment must be maintained indefinitely or the symptoms return. But this leaves the arthritic in no worse condition than the diabetic who must take insulin indefinitely. If the sufferer can prevent the agonizing symptoms of this extremely painful disease, he would surely be willing to swallow a few pills every day from now on.

For a long time, health seekers have been sure there is something extremely valuable in royal jelly, which is the food fed to the queen bee larva, causing her to hatch as a queen rather than a worker bee—an entirely different kind of bee. Scientists in many countries are studying royal jelly constantly, analyzing it and breaking it down into its parts, then testing these on animals. Now, because of the fine work of these three British scientists, we know that royal jelly contains a substance, which, when given along with pantothenic acid, helps the rheumatoid arthritis patient to use this vitamin correctly and hence to recover from symptoms of illness. And, from this research, we know that osteoarthritis patients can often gain relief of symptoms by taking the B vitamin along with another substance which apparently helps the body to use it.

We don't know whether this inability to use a B vitamin is inherited or occurs because of some other reason—years of eating improperly, for instance. Or, perhaps, it may be a much greater than average need for pantothenic acid over many years. Nor do we know how soon American doctors will try this form of treatment on their arthritis patients, who, at present, are generally told just to take aspirin and other painkillers for relief of their pain. What we do know is that, once again, natural foods and vitamins have shown to be curative, because a disease is apparently triggered by the body's misuse of a certain important nutrient. We can only hope that eventually scientists will finally unravel all of the complex threads of the various steps in digestion, assimilation and absorption, so that we can prevent conditions like arthritis before they arise.

In the meantime, arthritis sufferers continue to swallow tons of aspirin and aspirin compounds each year. According to the U. S. Department of Health, Education and Welfare, aspirin and its derivatives are used more by Americans than any other nonprescribed medicine. Aspirin can erode away the lining of the stomach and thus cause ulcers. It can be very toxic, especially among children.

Two other London doctors, writing in *Lancet* for October 26, 1963, also investigated the use of pantothenic acid in dealing with arthritis. They, too, found that the blood of people with arthritis contains considerably less of this B vitamin than that of healthy people. They found, in addition, that the lower the amount of pantothenic acid in the blood, the more severe were the symptoms of arthritis. Patients whose blood levels were lowest were bedridden and badly crippled.

Interestingly enough, they found that vegetarians (not vegans—but people who eat milk and eggs), had, generally, higher levels of pantothenic acid than people who consume meat every day in a well-balanced diet.

The doctors decided to inject the B vitamin into a group of arthritic patients every day. After seven days of injections, the patients' symptoms improved and their blood levels of pantothenic acid rose. There was no further improvement, however, even though the injections were continued for another three weeks. As soon as the injections stopped, the blood levels of the vitamin dropped again.

They also injected royal jelly into a group of arthritic patients every day for a month. There was no change in their condition. When they injected both royal jelly and the B vitamin, some of the patients improved—just like the previous studies we discussed—and their joints moved more easily. But the improvement was not permanent. When these same injections were given to arthritic vegetarians, symptoms disappeared rapidly and, in nine patients at least, the symptoms did not return. Some of the patients suffered from the injections and others did not improve, the doctors said. But they planned to continue their research.

From a Japanese journal, the *Tohoku Journal of Experimental Medicine* for November 25, 1961, we find that a survey of 200 Japanese showed that levels of pantothenic acid declined in the blood from the age of 30 on. And in the *Journal of Nutrition* for December 1961, we find that requirements for pantothenic acid may vary widely. Dr. Roger J. Williams and other researchers have always felt this to be true.

Writing in *Nutrition in a Nutshell*, Dr. Williams said: "Whether or not human beings are subject to pantothenic acid deficiency depends on how their needs compare quantitatively with the available supply. Wide distribution without regard to the quantities has nothing whatever to do with the question of human deficiencies. The quantitative aspects of nutrition are all important."

In other words, it does not matter how much pantothenic acid there is in the food you individually eat. If you happen to need far more than that, you are going to be deficient in this important vitamin. Dr. Williams says that, since human milk contains about 18 times more pantothenic acid than thiamine, it would seem that we need about 18 times more in our everyday meals. Although pantothenic acid is not destroyed to any extent in cooking, as some vitamins are, dry heat is very destructive of this B vitamin. So toasting bread causes a loss of pantothenic acid.

A Japanese medical journal reported in 1966 on an investigation of the diet in one region of Japan where the people eat "washed" rice as a staple. It was found that the blood of these people was lacking in pantothenic acid. Apparently it is washed away when the rice is processed. Looking further, the researchers discovered that these folks had higher blood pressure than people in other parts of Japan where the B vitamin is not lacking in the diet. Could it be that pantothenic acid is important in maintaining correct blood pressure? The Japanese doctors believe so.

German physicians, writing in *Deutsche Medi-*

zinische Wochenschrift, August 4, 1967, report that pantothenic acid was used to reduce "significantly" the toxic reactions of an antibiotic, kanamycin. This drug affects the ears unfavorably, as do some other antibiotics. Taking the B vitamin prevents some of this damage, the doctors said.

"Pantothenic acid deficiency, by itself, is probably uncommon in mental disease," said Dr. Roger J. Williams in his new book, *Nutrition Against Disease*. "Yet pantothenic acid is essential to brain functioning. Its lack can cause nerve degeneration in animals, and prisoners placed on a diet deficient in this vitamin apparently suffered from profound mental depression as a result. . . The fact that both animals and humans are reported to stand stress better when they are administered large doses of pantothenic acid is pertinent to this problem. Clearly, pantothenic acid is one more link in the nutritional chain needed to prevent mental disease."

Meanwhile, it is wise to guarantee as much of this important vitamin in your diet as possible, just in case you are one of the people whose requirement is high. The chart on page 240 shows the pantothenic acid content of some common foods. Why not list everything you ate today, then list its pantothenic acid content and total the amount. A day's menu of an orange and two eggs for breakfast, a cheese sandwich on whole wheat bread for lunch, and a dinner of roast beef, potatoes and vegetable, with, say, three cups of milk and three more slices of whole grain bread during the day, would give you less than 12 milligrams of pantothenic acid Officially no recommendation has been made for a daily intake of this B vitamin.

CHAPTER 9

Biotin

SCIENTISTS HAVE KNOWN for many years that a diet in which there are large amounts of uncooked egg white may bring about a deficiency in biotin. The reason for this is a protein—called avidin—which exists in raw egg whites. This substance latches onto the B vitamin biotin and makes it unavailable to the body. The individual who eats large amounts of raw eggs will probably become deficient in this vitamin. Cooking inactivates the aforementioned protein.

Such a case was seen by physicians at the Medical College of Birmingham, Alabama and reported in the *American Journal of Clinical Nutrition* for February 1968. A 62-year-old woman came to the hospital with alarming symptoms. She had no appetite, her mouth and lips were sore, she had a scaly dermatitis. Further, she suffered from nausea and vomiting, mental depression, pallor, muscle pains and pains around her heart. She also had tingling and pricking sensations in her hands and feet.

The doctors did the usual tests and found that she had anemia, abnormal heart action, extremely high cholesterol levels and certain liver symptoms. They asked her what she had been doing to get into this state. Here is her story.

She had suffered from cirrhosis, a kind of liver disorder probably brought on by rather heavy drinking earlier in life. Her doctor wanted her to get lots of excellent protein, so he told her to eat, every day, six raw eggs and two quarts of milk, in addition to her regular food. She did this for 18 months. After a few weeks on this diet, she lost her appetite, but, because she wanted to obey doctor's orders, she went o with the raw eggs and milk. She also took a vitamin capsule which the doctor had prescribed fo her, however, it contained no biotin. She als took several brewer's yeast tablets.

"Thus," said the authors of the article, "the stage was set for the development of biotin deficiency." Her symptoms developed rapidly and she was in serious condition when she came to the hospital. After they had taken her history, the doctors immediately tested her for biotin and found that she was deficient in this B vitamin. They gave her injections of biotin and within three days, all her symptoms began to disappear.

Because of this one B vitamin deficiency, the patient had a reddened, sore tongue. Her lips were full of slits and crusts. They occasionally bled. She had a tendency to bruise easily. She had difficulty in swallowing, along with nausea and vomiting. She felt tired, exhausted, out of breath all the time. She had a pain under her heart not related to eating but appeared to be relieved by belching. She had some abdominal swelling which eventually became severe. Two weeks before she came to the hospital, she developed swollen ankles.

When she was discharged, cured. she was told not to eat uncooked eggs and was placed on a high protein diet. Several months later she had great emotional stress when her husband died and she stopped eating the prescribed diet, developed a fever and cough and had trouble sleeping. When she came back to the hospital, the doctors gave her injections of biotin again and her symtoms disappeared.

There are three extremely important lessons to be learned from this story. First, although eggs are an excellent food and should be eaten daily, don't eat raw eggs in abundance. Obviously, six raw eggs per day is far more than anyone with any nutrition background would recommend. But don't shy away completely from eggs that you eat alone or use in cooking. There is still not enough evidence to show that the cholesterol in eggs is harmful, especially since eggs also contain lecithin, an emulsifier, which probably helps to break up the cholesterol so that it does not clog the arteries.

Second, when you are selecting food supplements, try to get those which contain the entire B Complex, even the obscure ones like biotin. You don't know what peculiar circumstances in your own daily life may be responsible for destroying or inactivating any given B vitamin, so it's good insurance to get them all. The lady was taking brewer's yeast and doesn't brewer's yeast contain biotin? Yes, it does. It contains all of the B vitamins. But, obviously, she was not getting enough biotin in her food, the vitamin capsule and the brewer's yeast.

Third, this patient began to suffer from biotin deficiency when she was under stress and was not eating properly. This would seem to indicate that she was one of those who, for some reason, needed more biotin than the rest of us.

The official booklet, *Recommended Dietary Allowances*, says this about biotin: "Daily needs are provided by diets containing 150 to 300 micrograms of biotin. This amount is provided by the average American diet." Obviously, this was not the case with the patient we have just discussed. This statement is also rather startling when you glance at the list of dietary sources of biotin on page 241.

Writing in *Chemical and Engineering News*, September 23, 1968, Cornell University scientists say they have discovered that biotin performs a physiological function which they had not known about before. Researchers had long suspected that the B vitamin was present in a certain enzyme (a chemical substance which manufactures an amino acid or form of protein). In this case, the amino acid is arginine, which is essential for human health.

The process by which this takes place is almost unbelievably complicated. The chemical formula for the process takes up the entire lower half of the page in the chemical magazine. However, the finding is important for biochemists to know. And it is important for health seekers to know, because it indicates, once again, that we are just beginning to unravel the extremely complex skeins of knowledge about things nutritional. There is not now and never will be a time when we can state, "Now we know all there is to know about such-and-such a vitamin." There will always be something new to discover, perhaps even new vitamins.

In the case of the *C&EN* research, only a great deal of future work will determine how important this discovery is for human health. For instance, the genes, which control our inherited characteristics, do so through enzymes. If one or another of these enzymes is absent or partially lacking in a new-born baby, there may be very serious, even fatal, consequences. So the presence of a B vitamin in an enzyme is an important finding.

Just what does biotin do? We are not quite sure of all of its functions. But it is involved in the biosynthesis (that is, the creation in the body) of various substances essential for health. Among these are the unsaturated fats, those substances which are believed to play an important role in keeping us safe from circulatory disorders, such as heart attacks.

It is believed that the normal human intestine contains bacteria which manufacture some biotin so that it is not necessary to get all of it that we need from food. But, of course, there are many people in whom these bacteria have been destroyed wholly or partially by various digestive disorders and by taking antibiotics which destroy bacteria wholesale—the harmful and the beneficial alike. It would certainly be wise, therefore, to get plenty of biotin with everyday meals, especially if you have, during your lifetime, taken large doses of antibiotics.

That biotin is destroyed or inactivated by a protein in egg white was discovered when scientists studied animals kept on a diet of nothing but raw egg white. The animals soon became ill and were restored to health only when ample amounts of biotin were included in their meals. A total deficiency of biotin has been induced in volunteers by feeding them a diet from which all the biotin was removed, then giving them large amounts of raw egg white. The consequences are immediately noticeable: a scaly dermatitis, a gray pallor, extreme fatigue, lack of appetite, muscle pains, insomnia, slight anemia and some heart problems.

In its July 3, 1971 issue, *Lancet* reports on the case of a 5-month-old infant brought to the hospital in serious condition. He suffered from persistent vomiting and an extensive skin rash. The rash had been present for some time and had been spreading, in spite of several drugs with which the physician tried to overcome it. The baby tended to vomit easily from birth. His breathing was abnormal and he appeared to have acidosis. His urine had a peculiar odor.

The doctors decided he was having trouble digesting protein. So they stopped all food and fed him intravenously. Then they began a series of elaborate tests. Just the description of the tests and their results takes up almost a page in the British medical journal. Although the words mean little to the average layman, the doctors found that the presence of certain substances in the child's urine suggested that the activity of a certain enzyme was impaired. Biotin works with this enzyme in the complex chemistry of the body, so the doctors gave the infant biotin.

First, they decided to put him back on protein food, and, when his condition was "stable," they would give him massive doses of biotin. Unfortunately, the food brought near disaster. The baby went into shock; the vomiting returned. So the doctors decided to give the biotin at once. "The effects both clinically and biochemically were impressive," the doctors stated. The vomiting stopped and the child's breathing became normal. His blood chemistry righted itself within a day. The skin rash disappeared and did not return. The baby became a happy, responsive, well child.

The doctors are sure, they tell us, that this child was born with impaired ability to deal with certain processes of digestion. The biotin righted the situation in his case. The researchers do not know, however, whether biotin will always cure such a condition in all children or whether it just happened this way for their little patient.

CHAPTER 10

Folic Acid

Folic acid—or folacin or pteroylglutamic acid—is one of the most interesting of the B group of vitamins because of a pecularity in its relationship with another B vitamin. In the little over 30 years since it was discovered, scientists have turned up an interesting complication between folic acid and vitamin B12. It seems they are very compatible. People who are suffering from a deficiency in folic acid may be helped considerably by very large doses of vitamin B12. But the condition is not completely cured until folic acid is given.

In cases of pernicious anemia, the disease of vitamin B12 deficiency, the victim is often found to be suffering from a deficiency of folic acid, as well. Disorders which interfere with the individual's ability to absorb food may possibly produce deficiency in both vitamins. Such disorders are sprue, celiac disease, any condition where vomiting or diarrhea are involved. Since folic acid is thought to be manufactured, to some extent, in the healthy intestinal tract, it is believed that taking antibiotics can destroy the bacteria which do this manufacturing. So people who have been taking these drugs by mouth for long periods of time may lack these two important B vitamins.

Also, there is apparently a very special need for folic acid in pregnancy. Some obstetricians feel that women should be tested for such deficiency before they become pregnant. Many doctors believe that the deficiency is widespread. Some doctors go so far as to say that folic acid deficiency is the No. 1 vitamin deficiency. Pregnant women with histories of abortion or miscarriage have been given folic acid to bring about a successful childbirth.

"Folic acid deficiency in pregnant women could well constitute a public health problem of dimensions we had not previously recognized," said Dr. A. Leonard Luhby and colleagues at New York Medical College. They are among the first to report a substantial number of patients with folic deficiency in early pregnancy. Of the 250 patients in all stages of pregnancy studied by the group, 55—or 22%—were folic acid deficient, Dr. Luhby said.

The potential health hazards of folic acid deficiency in both mothers and newborn babies are being investigated by Drs. Luhby, Martin L. Stone, Robert Feldman, Myron Gordon and Jack M. Cooperman, of the Department of Obstetrics and Gynecology and the Department of Pediatrics, New York Medical College Metropolitan Medical Center.

"In view of the fact that folic acid deficiency in mothers can produce damage to the fetus, resulting in abnormalities of development, it is particularly important that this deficiency be detected very early in pregnancy, when such damage is most likely to occur," Dr. Luhby added.

The New York researchers believe that deficiency of this vitamin in pregnant women in the U.S. is more prevalent than they previously thought. They have found that pregnant patients with a specially high risk for developing folic acid deficiency are those with toxemia, diabetes and hyperthyroidism. Also, the pregnant teenage girl who eats inadequately, and the older woman who has had many babies. In the survey they made, folic acid deficiency was three times as frequent among pregnant women with medical complications of pregnancy than those without such complications. Sixty percent of patients with toxemia of pregnancy and 60%

who developed abrupt separation of the placenta had low folic acid activity. The rate of the vitamin deficiency is 80% in twin and multiple pregnancies, the doctors stated.

Although poor eating habits play a significant role in folic acid deficiency in pregnancy, this is not the sole cause, Dr. Luhby and his associates found. They said that even the so-called good American diet may not always meet the folic acid requirements for pregnancy. To prevent possible complications, they urge an improved diet and vitamin supplementation early in pregnancy, especially in the high-risk patients.

Drs. Luhby and Cooperman have developed an invaluable aid to promptly detect a folic acid deficiency. The test checks the patient's urine for the presence of a substance called FIGLU (formiminoglutamic acid), which they say is an indicator of the level of folic acid enzymatic activity in cells.

According to a release from the U. S. Department of Agriculture, December 3, 1970, scientists at the University of California, Berkeley, working under a research grant from the Department, are trying to determine why some of the various chemical forms of folic acid in natural foods are more useful to the human body than others. The release mentions that "One in ten individuals examined in a recent National Nutrition Survey was found to have undesirably low levels of folic acid in the blood.

"The different chemical forms occurring in various foodstuffs cannot be used to equal advantage by the human body and are not as nutritionally available as folacin, an uncombined form of the vitamin," the USDA said. "Some individuals have developed folic acid deficiency on diets containing 200 to 500 micrograms of this nutrient per day, even though the recommended allowance for folacin (folic acid) established by the Food and Nutrition Board of the National Academy of Sciences as being adequate for persons in good health is only about 100 micrograms per day."

It is especially distressing to find, in the *Journal of the American Medical Association* for October 5, 1970, an article by a Florida physician who says that folic acid deficiency has been found among women taking oral contraceptives. It appears that the drug shuts off some mechanism which is essential for them to absorb the vitamin from food. Dr. Richard R. Streiff tells us of seven women who came to his clinic with anemia. They had been taking no drugs—except contraceptives—which they had been taking regularly for at least 1½ years. They had been eating good diets, he said, but their bone marrow showed evidence of megaloblastic anemia, which is the condition associated with serious lack of folic acid.

By complicated tests, this doctor discovered that the folic acid given these women in a dietary supplement was absorbed. But that form of the vitamin which appeared in food had to be processed by some body mechanism which apparently did not work when the women were taking The Pill.

In another article in the *Journal of the American Medical Association* (November 30, 1970), we are told of the families of three physicians—all quite affluent we might add—where the young daughters of the family suffered from lack of folic acid and were anemic. In every case the family was large and their eating habits were irregular, since the fathers had very irregular hours. Said the author, "Small families usually consume prepared meals together, whereas large families eat food which they select as individuals or in small groups. Frequently, this unsupervised diet . . . contains much carbohydrate, with few leafy vegetables and little protein. Since carbohydrate foods usually contain only small amounts of iron and folic acid, members of large families without organized eating habits may develop iron and folic acid deficiency."

In the *New England Journal of Medicine* for June 9, 1966, a Connecticut physician writes to complain about the fact that folic acid is usually not in nutritional supplements given to pregnant women. He tells of three women at his clinic suffering from megaloblastic anemia. One of them died. She had not sought the aid of a doctor during her pregnancy. Possibly a doctor would have discovered the deficiency and could have saved her life. In the same medical journal, for April 7, 1966, Dr. Mortimer S. Greenberg is quoted as saying that, although a considerable percentage of all young pregnant women may be deficient in folic acid, of 48 vitamin preparations listed in the Physicians' Desk Reference for use as supplements for pregnant women, "only five contain any folic acid."

The reason why folic acid is not permitted in considerable amounts in food supplements has to do, again, with its close relationship with vitamin B12. The disease pernicious anemia, which can be fatal, is caused by lack of vitamin B12. So closely is folic acid related to vitamin B12 that a fair amount of folic acid in the diet can mask the nervous system symptoms that may affect the pernicious anemia victim. So the disease may progress to the point where nerve tissue is seriously involved, without the patient or his doctor knowing that he is suffering from pernicious anemia. So food supplements sold without prescription are not permitted to contain more than 0.1 milligram of folic acid per day.

As you can see, this has nothing to do with

the wholesomeness and desirability of this essential B vitamin. We all need it. We must all get some of it every day, if we are to remain healthy. But we are not allowed to get more than a tiny amount in a food supplement because of the danger posed to that infrequent person who might be suffering from pernicious anemia. An effort is now being made by the American Medical Association Council on Foods and Nutrition to raise the amount of folic acid permitted in food supplements from 0.1 milligram to 0.4 milligram, because of newer methods of diagnosing pernicious anemia, which make unnecessary the present regulations in regard to folic acid.

Until this regulation is changed, we have no choice but to get plenty of folic acid at meals. It's not difficult if you are eating a highly nutritious diet, as we hope you are, for those foods which are richest in the other B vitamins—as well as many minerals—are also the foods in which folic acid is most abundant. They are: liver, dark green leafy vegetables (spinach, watercress, kale, parsley, escarole, etc.), asparagus, lima beans, whole grain cereals and breads and lentils. Please see the chart on page 242.

The importance of liver and whole-grain cereals and breads is once again highlighted here. White bread contains 15 micrograms of folic acid, compared to 27 for cracked wheat and 100 for a like amount of bran. A serving of liver contains 290 micrograms of folic acid, compared to only 5 for a hamburger.

Speaking before a Senate Committee on Nutrition and Related Needs on January 27, 1969, Dr. William Darby of the Vanderbilt School of Medicine said that "Colleagues of mine have repeatedly identified frank cases of deficiency states such as marasmus (starvation), nutritional anemias, scurvy and even beriberi in the wards of our hospital. Although the majority of these are medically conditioned deficiencies, practically all would have been prevented had the patients and their physicians utilized proper understanding of nutrition and diet."

Dr. Darby then related stories of official surveys which have turned up 616 cases of malnutrition, 15 of which had kwashiorkor (lack of protein) and 29 of marasmus. In another state there were evidences of low intakes or deficiencies of vitamin A and C; in another state of iron, vitamin A and folic acid.

Chromosomes are microscopic parts of cells which contain the genes by which heredity is determined. Damage to chromosomes has become one sympton by which doctors can diagnose certain diseases, such as mongolism. Now there is evidence, from a Public Health Service physician specializing in leukemia, that vitamins can repair chromosome damage.

Dr. Clark W. Heath reported in the magazine *Blood* that vitamin B12 and folic acid are involved in certain functions that go on in chromosomes, and lack of these vitamins may result in damage to the chromosomes. Fifteen patients were studied. Both blood and bone marrow cells showed damage to the chromosomes. After treatment with folic acid, vitamin B12, or both, the chromosomes returned to normal, he said.

A certain kind of anemia produced the most striking changes. Dr. Heath went on to say that a wide variety of medical findings are encountered in patients with deficiencies in folic acid and vitamin B12.

Two Soviet scientists reported treating psoriasis with folic acid, vitamin B12 and vitamin C. Working with 72 patients, they gave the injections twice daily for 20 days, then gave no treatment for three weeks, then injections again for 20 days.

Good results followed the first course of treatment in 29 patients, the second course in 25, and the third in four. Fourteen of the patients did not improve. Some of the patients had relapses later. Still, this would appear to be an area for researchers to pursue, hopefully to find a cure for this most distressing disorder.

In *Medical World News*, Dr. Myron Gordon, one of a team of pediatricians, is quoted as saying: "Some women may have a folic acid deficiency for months or even years, and it should be cleared up before they have children." Said the *News*, "With a carefully planned diet and vitamin supplements, adequate folic acid activity can rapidly be restored."

If these young, pregnant women have been suffering from a lack of folic acid for years, as Dr. Gordon suggests, they may also be suffering from lack of pyridoxine, PABA, choline, inositol, biotin and all the other B vitamins found in whole grains which are never restored in "enriched" flour and cereals. Wheat germ, incidentally, the little nutritious nubbin which is removed from cereals when they are refined, contains up to 160 micrograms of folic acid in one-fourth cup.

Another aspect of anemia during pregnancy was mentioned by Dr. C. R. Whitfield, writing in the *Journal of Obstetrics and Gynecology of the British Commonwealth.* On the staff of Queen's University in Belfast, Ireland, Dr. Whitfield said that a pregnant woman who is sensitive to gluten might develop megaloblastic anemia. He cautioned such women to shy away from wheat and flour products such as cakes, breads, cereals, spaghetti, pancakes, etc. In these cases, the gluten apparently causes the villi, or small threadlike projections in the small intestine, to atrophy and this interferes with the absorption of folic acid. In studying 36 pregnant women with this condition, Dr. Whitfield was able to bring improvement in most cases with a gluten-free diet and oral doses of folic acid.

Dr. Even Ludvig Stokstad, at the time with the University of California, is one of those scientists who believes that the commonest vitamin deficiency in the world is a deficiency in folic acid. This was brought out in the September 11, 1969 issue of *New Scientist*.

Said the article: "Folic acid is an essential vitamin for every living cell. It is normally in balance with vitamin B12 and, like it, can correct the pernicious form of anemia; but, unlike it, it can produce neurological symptoms such as degeneration of the spinal cord."

The problem in giving folic acid as a treatment for pernicious anemia is the matter of nerve involvement. It seems that, if the doctor gives folic acid to the pernicious anemia patient, this vitamin can cure all the symptoms of this serious disease except the nerve symptoms. These will progress at the same rate but the patient may be unaware of them until they have gone too far and it is too late to do anything about them. So the sensible thing appears to be to give both vitamins—folic acid and vitamin B12—along with a substance that seems to be essential for vitamin B12 to be absorbed by the digestive tract.

Medical World News indicates that other vitamins may be involved as well. This medical journal tells the pathetic story of a 3-year-old girl, the victim of diabetes and deafness, who developed pernicious anemia at the age of 11. Vitamin B12 and folic acid were both given by doctors at Duke University. There was no improvement. Then a multiple-vitamin, high-potency capsule was administered. And the little girl's anemia began to improve.

After the child was discharged, she was given no more vitamins of any kind and she had a relapse. Her insulin requirements had also gone up. She was again admitted to the hospital, where the doctors gave her large amounts of each of the vitamins in the multiple-vitamin capsule. They found that large amounts of thiamine brought about an improvement in her condition. She was sent home again, still with no vitamin supplementation. Again she relapsed. This time the doctors gave her 20 milligrams of thiamine a day and sent her home telling her family to continue this treatment. The child has had no relapses.

The doctors were puzzled as to why this particular B vitamin made such a difference. They concluded that "she has a defect in a single thiamine dependent enzyme and dietary amounts are insufficient to keep her from developing anemia, whereas superphysiologic amounts (that is, far more than the normal recommended amounts) corrected the situation."

The doctors do not know, they say, whether lack of thiamine had anything to do with her diabetes, her deafness or other things that were wrong with her. They fear, they explained, that their treatment was too late to reverse all these conditions, for too much damage had been done.

In addition to the cases we have mentioned, old folks, especially those living alone, are apt to neglect the foods which contain the most folic acid and the other B vitamins. Everyone should eat a nutritionally good diet every day. By this we mean plenty of the four essential groups of food: meat, fish, shellfish and poultry; vegetables and fruits; dairy products and eggs; whole grain cereals, nuts and seed foods like peanuts, sunflower seeds, soybeans, etc.

Then make it a habit to eat liver and/or some of the organ meats at least once a week; oftener if possible. If you and your family simply cannot stand liver, then get some desiccated liver, which contains everything in the original liver but the water. You can take the tablets or sprinkle desiccated liver into casseroles and other dishes.

Finally, don't make the mistake the Duke University doctors did when they took away the little girl's vitamin pills. You, too, may have excessive need for one or more of the B vitamins, vitamin C, etc. A high potency, one-a-day vitamin capsule is good insurance. Taking capsules or tablets of individual vitamins is even better.

According to *Recommended Dietary Allowances*, 7th Edition, 1968, the following amounts of folic acid are suggested: infants (0.05 to 0.1 milligram daily); children (0.1 to 0.3 milligram daily); males (0.4 milligram daily); females (0.4 milligram daily); pregnant women (0.8 milligram daily); lactating women (0.5 milligram daily).

CHAPTER 11

Vitamin B12

In an article in the *Journal of the American Medical Association* for June 23, 1968, it is stated that iron deficiency anemia plagues much of the world, especially the less prosperous nations. It was suggested by one South American health official that iron should be put into table salt, since this is the one seasoning that even very poor people in the tropics use. Other investigators recommended using soybean preparations—rich in iron, other minerals, protein and the B vitamins—as food supplements, especially among people whose diets consist largely of vegetables.

Another form of anemia—pernicious anemia—which is especially noticeable among teen-age girls, women and the elderly—can be cured with vitamin B12. Dr. E. Lester Smith, writing in the

June 11, 1964 issue of *New Scientist*, said: "The 5th of May is still celebrated as 'red crystal day' in my laboratory. That was the date in 1948 when the first microscopic crystals of vitamin B12 appeared. They had been isolated from liver." Dr. Smith is one of the world's foremost authorities on vitamin B12, which is also scientifically called cobalamine and cyanocobalamin.

Containing perhaps the most complex chemical formula of any vitamin, B12 is the only vitamin to contain a metal—cobalt—and also phosphorus. Wherever vitamin B12 is found in nature, its source is microorganisms—that is, bacteria of one kind or another, for only these lowly creatures are able to manufacture this vitamin. Unlike many vitamins, it cannot be duplicated synthetically in a laboratory. It is, therefore, the most potent of known vitamins. The daily human requirements amount to only a few micrograms.

We do not know how vitamin B12 acts in our bodies, but it is believed to be involved in the way we use protein, fats and carbohydrates. As we mentioned in another chapter, it performs some of its functions in connection with folic acid, but, as yet, we do not know too much about this association.

"Fortunately for those who need it, vitamin B12 does not have to be extracted from natural sources like liver . . . but is made by large scale fermentation procedures akin to those used for penicillin and other antibiotics," said Dr. E. Lester Smith. "It is really one of the cheapest vitamins reckoned by dose."

Pernicious anemia is a disease of the blood cells which is fatal if it goes untreated. Pernicious, of course, means "deadly" or "tending to be fatal." Until fairly recent times, no treatment was known. Then it was found that injections of liver extract cured the disease. More recently, as it was noted, it has been decided that the vitamin B12 in liver is the curative agent. Apparently there is a certain substance, called the "intrinsic factor," present in the normal stomach which allows the healthy person to absorb vitamin B12 from food. When this substance is lacking, the individual cannot absorb the B12. So he develops pernicious anemia. That is why injections of the vitamin are required for a cure. Taking it orally would not accomplish a cure, since it would not be absorbed. We are told, however, that large doses of the vitamin permit some of it to be absorbed, even in persons whose stomachs apparently lack the important "intrinsic factor."

Gastroenterology, the medical journal, reported in 1962 that laboratory rats on a diet deficient in iron soon lost their ability to absorb vitamin B12. It is also true that people suffering from some chronic condition that does not permit them to absorb their food properly will almost inevitably be lacking in vitamin B12. This, of course, refers to those who have diarrhea, dysentery, sprue, and people who have had part of their stomachs removed.

Since vitamin B12 exists almost exclusively in foods of animal origin—meat, fish and milk—it is not surprising that vegans (those who eat only foods of vegetable origin) may suffer from a lack of vitamin B12. This is not because they lack the ability to absorb the vitamin; it just isn't present in their food. However, the companion vitamin, folic acid, is found in vegetables, grains and fruits, so the vegan usually does not suffer from some of the symptoms of pernicious anemia, which folic acid can control. Unfortunately, the more serious symptoms, which involve actual deterioration of the nerves and the brain, may be going on silently and becoming worse with every passing year. The vegan, therefore, may find himself eventually with a quite serious case of pernicious anemia which could have been prevented easily, even on a totally vegetarian diet, by taking vitamin B12 in extremely small amounts.

The nervous and mental symptoms accompanying vitamin B12 deficiency are so common that medical journals are quite concerned about them. Here's a comment from *Lancet*, October 9, 1965: "It is now generally recognized that vitamin B12 deficiency may be present with a wide variety of psychiatric (that is mental illness) manifestations and without anemia or gross neurological (nerve damage) signs; and that these may precede the physical disturbances by months or years." This London physician went on to recommend that all patients admitted to mental hospitals be tested for vitamin B12 deficiency, even if they showed no signs of anemia. And the *Journal of the American Medical Association,* October 11, 1965, stated in an editorial, "Although vitamin B12 deficiency is now well recognized and both the (blood) and (nerve) symptoms respond to treatment with cyanocobalamin, patients with this deficiency are still common."

How much vitamin B12 do you need every day and how can you be sure you are getting it? The Food and Nutrition Board lists the following Recommended Dietary Allowances:

Infants—1.0 to 2 micrograms
Children—2 to 5 micrograms
Males—5 to 6 micrograms
Females—5 to 6 micrograms
Pregnancy—8 micrograms
Lactation—6 micrograms

Pernicious anemia patients sometimes receive injections of 100 micrograms daily, although injected doses of as much as 30,000 micrograms have been given without any unpleasant reactions.

The Canadian Medical Association stated in the December 12, 1964 issue of its *Journal* that they believe that only one to three micrograms daily are necessary for vegans to keep their stores of vitamin B12 up where they belong. So it would seem that most of us do not need more than that amount, unless we are suffering from an absorption problem. In that case, a doctor should be prescribing vitamin B12.

In *Let's Get Well*, Adelle Davis says that she believes strict vegetarians who eat no food from animal sources should probably take 50 micrograms of vitamin B12 each week "while their stomach secretions are still normal." She also suggests that, of vegetable foods, only yeast, wheat germ and soybeans contain appreciable traces of vitamin B12.

Liver, of course, contains the most vitamin B12. It is, therefore, suggested that everyone eat liver often. Its vitamin B12 content is only one of the near-miracle ingredients in this excellent food. It is fantastically rich in other B vitamins, along with many valuable minerals, including iron and copper.

There are many articles in medical journals and books on how valuable vitamin B12 is in dealing with other disorders. It has been used with some success in treating neuralgias and neuritis. It has also been used for bursitis. One doctor reports excellent results using vitamin B12 for psoriasis. He used 30 injections of 1,000 micrograms each before results were obtained. He reported on this experiment in the *British Medical Journal* for January 12, 1963. In all cases, the vitamin is being used as a drug —that is, in amounts which have no relation to the minimum daily requirement or the amounts you might get in food. We have no explanation as to why the vitamin produced results. Indeed, some critics say the improvement was not the result of the vitamin—any injection would have produced improvement. We do not know.

What we do know is that vitamin B12 is an important weapon in your arsenal against disease. You need it in extremely small amounts, but you absolutely must get those small amounts in your food. Nothing else can substitute for "the red vitamin." Of course, the health seeker has long recognized, merely as insurance against a deficiency, the necessity for taking vitamin B12 supplements, desiccated liver or even the entire B Complex tablets. The latter, when combined with vitamin C, are often suggested by dentists for good teeth and gum health.

In the October 1965 issue of *Archives of Neurology*, Dr. R. F. Mayer describes patients who had past or present deficiency in vitamin B12 to whom he gave tests of nerve function. At the same time, he tested other patients who did not have this deficiency. Dr. Mayer found that the farthest ends of the nerves may be affected by the vitamin B12 deficiency, although the nearer portion of the nerve remains healthy. In a few patients the nerve function returned to normal when they took vitamin B12 for six to 12 months.

Glaucoma is a serious eye condition which, if left untreated, may result in blindness. It is caused by the retention of fluids within the cavity of the eye, which exert pressure on the delicate lining. Russian researchers reported in 1961 and 1963 on treating this condition by injecting vitamin B12. They gave a daily dose of one-tenth of a milligram to 46 patients and obtained improvement in about half of the patients.

A Japanese physician has confirmed the Russian findings by giving one milligram of vitamin B12, injected twice a week for one month. The sight of seven of the affected 17 eyes improved, 10 gained in their field of vision, 10 showed a drop in pressure in the eye, and 13 improved in other ways. This is apparently an example of how a vitamin can be used as a drug, for there is no indication that glaucoma is caused by lack of vitamin B12 in the diet. Since the treatment is harmless and inexpensive, we wish American physicians would try it. The report that we have just discussed appeared in *New Scientist* for August 13, 1964.

Many of the women who long for children

without being able to conceive may be suffering from a lack of vitamin B12. Researchers at the Royal Infirmary in Glasgow, Scotland have found that women who could not have children for many years became pregnant when pernicious anemia was diagnosed and they were given injections of B12. One woman, for example, who married at 25, remained childless for 11 years, although no cause could be found for her infertility. Then she developed the symptoms of pernicious anemia—fatigue and a tingling in the hands and feet. She was given B12 therapy and became pregnant 11 months later.

If ordinary anemia, caused by lack of iron, were responsible for infertility, said the doctors, 10% of all women would be unable to have children, since that many suffer from iron deficiency anemia. But pernicious anemia is much more difficult to diagnose. It, therefore, goes undetected for years, until the telltale symptoms of an advanced case appear.

A physician in the Department of Pathology of the Royal Berkshire Hospital in Reading, England conducted a significant investigation of the relationship between vitamin B12 and sterility. He reported on his findings in the September 29, 1962 issue of *Lancet.*

Laboratory technicians assess a man's potential for fathering children by studying the condition of the sperm—the microscopic reproductive cell in the human semen which unites with the female reproductive cell to form the beginning of a new life. In cases where the complaint is sterility—or an inability to father children—the tiny sperm cells are generally found to be too few in number, unhealthful, or perhaps quite motionless, and, hence lifeless.

It has been found that, when some of the millions of sperm cells are formed abnormally, there is also a decrease in the total number of sperm cells and in the number of cells that appear to be alive. So, said Dr. Alan A. Watson, it is believed that perhaps the sperm cells are not maturing normally. Cells, of course, mature just as larger organisms do, and a cell which does not completely mature cannot function normally.

A veterinary doctor, writing in a breeder's journal, has shown that the fertility of sperm being used for artificial insemination of cattle improved when vitamin B12 was added to it. Deciding that there might be some connection between vitamin B12 levels and sterility in human sperm, Dr. Watson tested 30 patients at a sterility clinic. He checked the vitamin B12 level in the sperm and compared it to that of the blood. The B12 level in the sperm of two persons who were known to be fertile was found to be higher than the blood levels. In cases where the sperm of the patient was found to be abnormal—in other words, the cells were not normally formed—the vitamin B12 levels in the sperm were less than that of the blood.

Three of these had an absence of sperm or a serious lack of vitality in the remaining sperm. Dr. Watson believes that these tests show that vitamin B12 may be very intimately involved with the maturing of sperm cells. This seems to indicate that its presence or deficiency would be an important consideration in the treatment of sterility.

Commenting on Dr. Watson's findings in a later issue of *Lancet* (October 13, 1962), Doctors A. A. Sharp and L. J. Witts of Oxford, England describe the case of a patient of theirs—a man of 35 whose marriage had been childless. The sperm cells of this patient showed no activity, so they would be unable to fertilize an egg cell. In addition, it was found that many of the cells were improperly formed.

When they did further tests on this patient, the doctors found that his blood condition was very bad and he was suffering from pernicious anemia. He was given injections of B12 and the level of the vitamin in his blood rapidly returned to normal. Six months later, examination of the sperm showed that 75% were active and healthy. The sperm were also normally formed. Eighteen months after he had begun treatment, his wife had a healthy child.

It is well known to blood specialists, said the doctors, that women who have developed pernicious anemia during the reproductive period quite often conceive when they are given vitamin B12 to treat the anemia, even though they have been childless before this. They suggested that, whenever the sperm cells appear to be defective, physicians should test the level of B12 in the blood to see if pernicious anemia is present.

According to an article in the *Canadian Medical Association Journal* for May 12, 1962, inability to absorb vitamin B12 may be inherited. Surveys have shown that pernicious anemia seems to run in families, it was stated. More recently, in the *New England Journal of Medicine* for March 25, 1971, Graham H. Jeffries, M.B., Ch.B., said that "the intestinal absorption of physiologic amounts of vitamin B12—about 1 microgram daily—depends on a complex sequence of events in the gastrointestinal tract." He also said that "In the current issue of the *Journal,* Toskes et. al. present data suggesting that pancreatic exocrine secretions (external secretion from the pancreas) may participate in vitamin B12 absorption. Of 22 patients with pancreatic exocrine insuffiency, nine exhibited subnormal vitamin B12 absorption on Schilling tests." Jeffries concluded thusly: "The existence of a gastric factor necessary for normal vitamin B12 absorption was discovered by William Castle 43 years ago, but the total picture of that absorption still appears incomplete."

Says the National Academy of Sciences: "A mucoprotein secreted by the stomach, the intrinsic factor, appears to bind vitamin B12 and, with calcium, attaches the vitamin to the wall of the ileum (the last division of the small intestine), through which it is absorbed. It is transported bound to serum proteins and is stored primarily in the liver and, to some extent, in the kidney."

In *Nutrition Against Disease*, Dr. Roger J. Williams has this to say: "Vitamin B12 is definitely a link in the nutritional chain that protects against mental disease. In pernicious anemia, the mental symptoms are by no means uniform; they can range from such mild symptoms as having difficulty in concentrating or remembering to stuporous depression, severe agitation, hallucinations, or even manic or paranoid behavior.

"Like the symptoms in pellagra," continued Dr. Williams, "those caused by B12 deficiency may be very similar to those observed in schizophrenia. Yet the relationship between pernicious anemia and B12 is not simple; other factors may be involved as well. Sometimes administering B12 will clear up the mental symptoms associated with pernicious anemia rather slowly—

and, occasionally, incompletely. The relationship between vitamin and disease is not as direct as in the case of pellagra."

While the scientists continue to unravel the mysteries of B12, be certain that you are getting enough of it for your own mental and physical well being.

CHAPTER 12

Choline

FOR MANY YEARS, nutrition scientists have been calling choline (pronounced ko′lin) a B vitamin. The official booklet, *Recommended Dietary Allowances,* lists it among the B Complex, but does not make any recommendations for how much we should get every day. Says the booklet, "Choline is generally considered to be an essential nutrient in the diet. Choline deficiency has not been demonstrated in man, however, at any stage of life, and whether or not it is an essential dietary nutrient for man is unknown."

We do know, however, that it exists, along with other members of the B Complex, in foods in which this complex is plentiful. We know also that choline is essential in the diet of many animals and birds, where it protects them against abnormalities in pregnancy and lactation, anemia, cardiovascular disease and muscular weakness.

Under the right conditions, choline can apparently be manufactured by the human digestive tract—if there is enough of all the elements necessary to make it. These include an amino acid or form of protein, methionine (pronounced me-thi'o-nin), plus folic acid and vitamin B12, and a number of other ingredients. Of course, it seems possible that some condition of ill-health might make this process impossible. And, too, some common American diets will certainly not provide enough of all these essential ingredients.

What are some of the functions of this vitamin in the human body? As long ago as 1950, scientists discovered that rats, completely deprived of choline, developed high blood pressure. Adding choline to the diet lowered the pressure at once. Other scientists discovered that, by keeping rats on a diet in which there was just enough choline to keep them alive, they could produce cancer in about two-thirds of all the rats involved.

In the January 1950 issue of the *Proceedings of the Society of Experimental Biology and Medicine*, L. M. Morrison and W. F. Gonzales discuss the effective use of choline in certain heart cases. And in the *Journal of the American Medical Association* for September 16, 1950,

Italian researchers reported on the favorable use of choline in treating 14 women and one girl with hyperthyroid conditions. Three patients who had serious cases of the disorder were treated effectively with choline hydrochloride and 150,000 units of vitamin A. This combination was administered every five days for two- or three-week periods.

In 1951, Brown University scientists deprived rats of both protein and choline and produced liver cancer in animals which were not bred to be susceptible to the disease. Also in 1951, as reported in *Deutsche Medizinische Wochenschrift* (February 16), choline was used by German researchers to treat hepatitis. The choline reduced the duration of virus hepatitis by about one-half, the scientists reported.

Choline was used by a California group of researchers to prevent complications from artery hardening in humans. After about three years, fatalities from circulatory disorders were far lower in the group which had been taking choline every day. At the University of Toronto, as reported in *Science* for June 11, 1954, it was established that choline was important to the heart and blood vessel system in young rats.

Liver cirrhosis is a serious, sometimes fatal disease which doctors believe may be related to excessive drinking or harmful drugs, among other things. In laboratories, the condition can be induced in rats by feeding them a certain diet. The diet is low in protein and choline. In only five months, the cirrhosis appears.

Bicknell and Prescott, in *Vitamins in Medicine,* tell us that choline is essential for the correct use of fatty food by the body. Thus, liver damage is prevented. Choline is also essential for the proper use of cholesterol in the body. This is the fatty substance we have been warned against in recent years as a threat to circulatory health. Perhaps we have somehow lost the ability to manufacture choline internally, or, perhaps, we have managed to pervert and disorder the elements in our processed food so thoroughly that we have destroyed those things in our food which our bodies need to manufacture choline. There seems to be little hope of turning up this kind of evidence in today's diet survey, where individual peculiarities in eating are hidden in the "averages" which are reported.

Let's say you're on a typical reducing diet. You're taking black coffee and grapefruit for breakfast, a dab of cottage cheese for lunch, and a bit of meat and salad without dressing for dinner. Choline appears, along with the other B vitamins, in food which is almost wholly absent from such a deficient diet. The less protein you eat, the less methionine you will have. You will recall this is the form of protein which is essential for the body to manufacture choline.

In *Nutrition Against Disease,* Dr. Roger J. Williams reports: "It has been found that rats can be induced to develop cancers if they are fed diets deficient in choline. In one experiment, 14 out of 18 rats developed cancers on the deficient diet, while no rats had cancers when the diet was supplemented with 0.2% choline.

"From these experiments," said Dr. Williams, "it cannot be concluded that choline is the only nutrient to be watched in connection with cancer prevention. It is not that simple. In these particular rats, choline may have been a limiting factor, but in other animals or human beings some other nutrient or nutrients might play a comparable role."

In *Let's Get Well,* Adelle Davis has given us a great deal of information about choline, for she has done a thorough job of studying all the medical and scientific literature available. She tells us of the protection given to the liver by choline and vitamin E, when a high-fat diet is eaten by laboratory animals. In diets deficient in both choline and protein (diets which contain lots of alcohol, for example), the liver can be badly damaged.

Perhaps most important is the effect of lack of choline on cholesterol levels in the blood. Lecithin is a substance which the body manufactures when there is enough choline present, along with another B vitamin, inositol. The lecithin apparently keeps cholesterol in such an emulsified state that it does not settle on artery walls or collect as gall bladder stones. Eggs are especially rich in lecithin, as well as methionine, so eggs remain one of our most valuable foods, even for people with hardening of the arteries and heart problems.

Says Miss Davis: "When patients recovering from heart attacks received daily 2,000 and 750 milligrams of choline and inositol respectively, the size of the cholesterol particles and the amount of fat in the blood quickly decreased; two months later the blood cholesterol had dropped to normal. Blood lecithin has also increased and cholesterol been reduced after choline has been given."

Adelle Davis tells us also that deficiencies in choline may be responsible for high blood pressure in people suffering from diabetes, overweight, nephritis (a kidney disorder) or heart disease. She points out that alcohol causes the need for choline to increase, and that alcohol causes a rapid rise in fatty substances in the blood. Speaking of reducing diets, she reminds us that the major function of lecithin is to burn fat, so all the ingredients from which the body manufactures lecithin must be present in any successful reducing diet. These are choline, pyridoxine, inositol, plus one of the unsaturated fats and the mineral magnesium. Such research indicates, she says, that "it is not entirely the amount of food eaten that causes obesity, but the lack of nutrients required to convert the fat into energy." And choline is one of these.

How can you be sure you are getting enough choline? You can be sure if you are getting enough of all those foods in which the entire B Complex is most abundant: meat, fish, poultry, eggs, wholegrains, green leafy vegetables, seeds of all kinds. The best sources of B vitamins in foods and food supplements are, of course, wheat bran, wheat germ and brewer's yeast.

We cannot end a discussion of choline without talking more about lecithin. Lecithin (pronounced less'-i-thin) is that emulsifying substance which apparently breaks cholesterol down into tiny droplets so that it cannot damage the inside walls of arteries. As we have seen, choline is one of the ingredients of lecithin. So by using lecithin as a supplement, you can increase your intake of choline as well as guaranteeing a better metabolism of fats in your body chemistry.

The richest natural sources of lecithin are eggs and soybeans. So, apparently, eggs, which are rich in cholesterol, are also filled wtih the substance which renders it harmless in arteries. Soybeans are vegetable foods so they contain no cholesterol. But they contain so much lecithin that they are usually the source for the food supplements you may be using: lecithin flakes, granules, liquid lecithin, etc. You can use these in any appropriate dish: a teaspoon or so in an omelet, or salad dressing, soup or stew.

"Dietary choline protects against poor growth, fatty liver development, and renal (kidney) damage in many experimental animals, and against perosis, or slipped tendon, in the fowl," says the National Academy of Sciences. "Also, it has been reported to protect against abnormalities in pregnancy and lactation in the rat and mouse, anemia in the guinea pig, rat and dog, cardiovascular disease in the rat, and muscular weakness in the guinea pig and rabbit."

There is no doubt that, as more research is completed, choline will be determined even more important to the good health of man.

CHAPTER 13

Inositol

IN THE EARLIER DAYS of vitamin research, inositol was called a B vitamin and investigated as such. Today, it is not mentioned in the official booklet which sets standards for the amounts of the different vitamins and minerals which are considered officially to be essential to human life. So, perhaps, we might say that inositol (pronounced i-nō′si-tol′) is a substance which appears with all the other B vitamins in those foods in which the B group is abundant, and let it go at that.

But one aspect of the physiology of this vitamin-like substance worries us to such an extent that we are unwilling to dismiss it quite so easily. *Vitamins in Medicine*, the classic book on vitamins by Franklin Bicknell and Frederick Prescott, tells us that lindane, one of the common pesticides, is believed to kill insects by destroying the inositol in their bodies.

In *Silent Spring,* Rachel Carson recites the list of grievances any sensible person should have against lindane. She says, "We can hang strips impregnated with the chemical lindane in our closets and garment bags or place them in our bureau drawers for a half-year's freedom from worry over moth damage. The advertisements contain no suggestion that lindane is dangerous. Neither do the ads for an electronic device that dispenses lindane fumes—we are told that it is safe and odorless. Yet the truth of the matter is that the American Medical Association considers lindane vaporizers so dangerous that it conducted an extended campaign against them in its *Journal.*"

Miss Carson tells us that lindane is stored in the brain and liver and may induce profound and long lasting effects on the central nervous system. Plants treated with lindane became monstrously deformed with tumor-like swellings on their roots. Their cells grew in size, being swollen with chromosomes which doubled in number. The doubling continued in future divisions until further cell division became mechanically impossible. She tells us that a Mayo Clinic expert reports that patients admitted with diseases of the blood-forming organs (leukemia and related conditions), almost without exception, have had a history of exposure to various toxic chemicals, among them the pesticide lindane.

Scientists have known since 1948 that lindane destroys inositol in living tissues. Doesn't it seem almost impossible to believe that they could have continued to allow us to use this pesticide all these years without one single warning of its potential for harm?

There is no way for you to know how many times you have been exposed to lindane even if you yourself never use pesticides of any kind. In the days when lindane vaporizers appeared in almost every public place, all of us got a dose of this poison. Does the rising rate of many assorted diseases have anything to do with this exposure? There is no way of knowing. Toxic substances are all around us in our modern technological society. Since the publication of *Silent Spring,* we are a bit more careful about pesticides. Government regulations are a bit more strict.

Inositol is closely related in function to the B vitamins choline and biotin. Bicknell and Prescott tell us that rats deprived of inositol lose their hair. Other animals develop severe digestive troubles when the inositol is removed from their food. Adelle Davis tells us *(Let's Get Well)* that both the B vitamin choline and inositol are necessary for the body to manufacture lecithin.

Patients recovering from heart attacks who were given large amounts of choline and inositol showed rapid decrease of the fatty substances in their blood. Within two months the cholesterol levels had dropped to normal.

In 1950 experiments with rabbits given cholesterol showed that, when inositol was given along with the fatty substance, the blood levels of cholesterol did not soar as they might be expected to do in a rabbit, whose natural diet does not contain cholesterol.

Dr. Walter Eddy in his book *Vitaminology* mentions a curious fact about the possible relation of inositol deficiency and drinking too much coffee. When laboratory animals were given large amounts of caffeine, a paralysis occurred which could be cured by giving them inositol. So possibly caffeine may have some destructive effect on this vitamin-like substance —something to keep in mind when you are debating whether to go on drinking coffee or switch to one of the caffeine-free kinds or one of the fine herb teas.

Inositol is available in food along with other members of the B complex of vitamins—meats, fish, poultry, organ meats, leafy green vegetables, seeds and wholegrain cereals, nuts, wheat germ, brewer's yeast, also in many fruits and vegetables. It is noteworthy that, among the organ meats, inositol is very abundant in heart muscle. It is axiomatic that those organs in which vitamins or minerals are stored have special need for those nutrients. So it seems that inositol may be very important for a healthy heart. That's nothing to be ignored these days when heart disease is our leading cause of death. Get plenty of inositol in those foods in which it occurs. You can also obtain it in natural food supplements where it occurs along with other important and essential members of the B complex of vitamins.

CHAPTER 14

Para-amino-benzoic Acid (PABA)

THE B VITAMIN with the tongue-twister name, Para-amino-benzoic acid, is not listed as a vitamin in the official handbook *Recommended Dietary Allowances.* But its use in human nutrition has been long and interesting. Mostly it has been associated with skin welfare and graying hair. Nobody is quite sure why or how it acts in the body.

We call it PABA for short. Drs. Bicknell and Prescott in their massive book *The Vitamins in Medicine*, tell us that PABA is unique in that it is a vitamin within a vitamin. It seems that it is part of folic acid. When sulfanilamide, the antibiotic, first came into use in the 1940's, it was found that its chemical formula is very much like that of PABA. So when people or experimental animals were given the drugs internally the PABA in their intestines counteracted it, so that it became ineffective.

Early in research work with PABA, scientists discovered that, when they withheld it from the diet of laboratory animals, their hair became white. It was believed that PABA was essential for the synthesis of folic acid in the intestinal tract and the lack of folic acid was the real reason for the white hair.

At any rate, people with prematurely white hair wanted to know if lack of PABA was the reason for their loss of pigment and if they might be able to restore the color if they took PABA. One researcher claimed that he could restore lost hair color by giving massive doses of PABA over long periods of time.

Adelle Davis, in *Let's Get Well*, tells us that she has seen many instances of gray hair which returned to its original color temporarily, but it quickly became gray again "unless one continues to eat yogurt, liver, yeast and wheat germ. Persons who take 5 milligrams of folic acid and 300 milligrams of PABA and pantothenic acid daily with some B vitamins from natural sources can usually prevent hair from graying and often restore its color."

Unfortunately, both PABA and folic acid are

restricted by the FDA to very small amounts in food supplements. In the case of folic acid it is because of this vitamin's close relationship with vitamin B12, which we discussed earlier. In the case of PABA, doctors used to worry about the fact that it makes sulfanilimide ineffective. These days this drug is used very seldom, so there seems to be no point to the restriction. PABA is available on doctors' prescription and it is also sold in supplement form.

Dr. Frank A. Evans tells us, in *Diseases of Metabolism,* that falling hair has been reported by some obese woman after several months on an extremely restricted diet—a daily intake of 350 to 450 calories. These diets were high in protein and were not apparently diets which would lead to gross deficiencies in any nutriment. Yet the reducers lost large amounts of hair. PABA was given and the hair grew in again.

"Results have been satisfactory and its continued use is recommended," Dr. Evans said.

The following B vitamins, incidentally, have been studied in relation to hair, both in regard to baldness and hair color: riboflavin, biotin, pyridoxine, PABA and pantothenic acid. The last two appear to be related to one another in their effect on hair health, according to Dr. Thèrése Terroine, writing in *Vitamins and Hormones* (Vol. 18, 1960).

In 1941, Dr. Benjamin Sieve reported on very encouraging work recoloring gray hair with PABA. He claimed beneficial results in 82% of 460 patients, as reported in *Vitamins and Hormones, II.*

In 1942, Banay discussed his work with 20 prisoners to whom he gave 100 milligrams of PABA three times daily for six to eight months. He says there was progressive darkening of hair, beginning at the back and working forward in geometric designs, with patches or islands of dark hair showing up among the gray. In 1943, Dr. H. Brandaleone reported in the conservative *Proceedings of the Society of Experimental Biology and Medicine* (Vol. 53, p. 47) that he had had success giving brewer's yeast along with pantothenic acid.

Seven of his patients took 100 milligrams of pantothenic acid, plus 200 milligrams of PABA, plus 50 grams of brewer's yeast daily. A second group took the brewer's yeast and the PABA, and a third group took yeast and pantothenic acid. He reported that two of the patients receiving PABA with yeast showed a definite return of hair coloring within three months.

The *Journal of the American Medical Association*, commenting on the subject of vitamins for gray hair in 1943, mentioned this experiment favorably, then went on to say, "It is already apparent, however, that much of the publicity concerning anti-gray hair factors has left a distorted impression."

With this discouraging official pronouncement, reports on experiments of this kind are rare in today's scientific journals. The only exception is research on gray hair among animals which have commercial value, such as sheep.

Copper, the trace mineral, is extremely important for the health of several kinds of animals. Great losses were suffered by wool growers when there was a deficiency of copper in the soil. The sensitivity of wool to lack of copper is so great that the wool of black sheep turns gray, even when there is no other symptom of copper deficiency. Adding copper to the diet turns the wool black once more. Taking the copper away brings graying once more.

Dr. E. J. Underwood, in *Trace Minerals in Human and Animal Nutrition*, tells us that apparently copper and pantothenic acid are related in their action on hair color. Perhaps, he says, one must have pantothenic acid in the diet to permit the copper to form the pigment that colors hair or wool.

The other field in which PABA has been recently shown to be almost a wonder drug is in the prevention of damage from sunburn. Way back in the 1940's scientists were finding they could prevent serious burns from the sun and from sunlamps by putting a PABA lotion on the exposed skin. And sure enough, it worked. We have no idea why it took so long for scientists to rediscover this important fact. That's the way things work out in the field of vitamin research. For years we got along with sunburn lotions which accomplished little or nothing.

In Spring of 1969 we began to get enthusiastic reports from scientists that they found PABA to be a "superior" sunscreen agent. Three scientists from the University of Pennsylvania told the Society of Cosmetic Chemists that they were getting far better results using PABA lotion than any of the commonly available suntan lotions could give.

Then several Boston doctors developed another formula which they claimed would screen out the ultraviolet rays of the sun "to provide protection from sunburn, skin cancer and aging of the skin." The formula was effective whether you used it at the seashore, the desert or the mountains. They mixed the vitamin with ethyl alcohol and tested it on prisoners in Arizona under the hot, dry sunshine there. The formulas used and all the scientific information about the tests appeared in the *New England Journal of Medicine* for June 26, 1969.

Bicknell and Prescott describe many more experimental uses of PABA in diseases where skin problems are involved. It has been used in massive doses to treat lymphoblastoma cutis, lupus erythematosus, scleroderma, pemphigus, and dermatitis herpetiformis. No one knows what causes any of these conditions or why PABA was effective in relieving them. But pictures in the book show clear improvement in the skin condition so long as the vitamin was being taken, and in massive doses.

PABA has also been used in the treatment of several diseases like Rocky Mountain Spotted Fever and certain kinds of typhus. It seems that this characteristic may become more important as cases of Rocky Mountain Fever become more common due to tick bites.

Adelle Davis tells us that PABA has also been used to treat vitiligo, the skin condition where pigment is lost, leaving large patches of entirely white skin. She tells us that pantothenic acid has also been used in massive doses to bring the color back to these unsightly patches of skin. PABA applied in an ointment has produced good results. Says Miss Davis, "I once told a 30-year-old woman with severe vitiligo that liver would probably help her more than any other food. A week later she joyously returned to show me that not a trace of it remained, but she had eaten ¼ pound of raw liver, frozen, diced and covered with catsup, at each meal. Several other persons have had the condition clear up slowly on a more appetizing diet."

The best sources of the vitamin PABA are

those same foods in which all the other B vitamins are most abundant: meat (especially organ meats like liver,) seeds of all kinds and unrefined cereals of all kinds, nuts, leafy green vegetables, brewer's yeast, wheat bran, wheat germ. Be sure to get enough of it.

CHAPTER 15

More Important Research with The B Complex

ONE OF THE most dramatic uses of a B vitamin to alleviate suffering was told at the "Conference on Aging" held March 6, 1972 in New York and already referred to. Dr. Abram Hoffer, who is President of the Huxley Institute for Bio Social Research, and, as we have mentioned, one of the world's leading nutritionists, told about the misfortunes of a group of 2,000 Canadian Army men who were sent in 1940 to help the British defend Hong Kong against the Japanese.

The entire contingent was promptly captured by the Japanese and put into the prisoner-of-war camp, where they remained for 44 months. "Most of the men who survived—and there was a fantastically high death rate—came out having lost one-third of their body weight and they had in the meantime suffered pellagra, beriberi, many infections and just about every deficiency disease known," Dr. Hoffer said.

The survivors were brought back to Canada in hospital ships, hospitalized and given what were then considered massive doses of vitamins. For example, 50 milligrams of niacin a day.

"These Hong Kong Veterans have since remained a perpetual problem to the Government of Canada," Dr. Hoffer said. "They are complaintive, neurotic. They never seem to do well."

Dr. Hoffer then told of one of the group, a friend of his, who suffered continued depression, fatigue, arthritis, neuritis—and, like the rest, was continuously making commission and pension demands on the government. Each morning it took the combined efforts of his wife and himself for one hour to get him out of bed so that he could become mobile, Dr. Hoffer said.

In 1960, Dr. Hoffer asked the man if he would object to some research on the effect of large doses of nicotinic acid (niacin) at the Geriatric Center where the doctor was then working. Although the two men were friends, the veteran had never been one of Dr. Hoffer's patients. At the time, therefore, Dr. Hoffer did not know the complete case history of his patient.

Dr. Hoffer started his patient on 3 grams of nicotinic acid a day and, within two weeks, the man had recovered and since that time he has remained well, with the exception of a period of two years when he went climbing the Rocky Mountains and forgot to take his vitamins with him, Dr. Hoffer said.

After the mountain climb, the patient noticed that, within two weeks, his joints were beginning to freeze; his cold intolerance was beginning to come back; his neuritis was coming back; and he was becoming once more very depressed and tense.

"He has never made this experiment again and has remained well until this day," Dr. Hoffer continued. "In fact, while in Hawaii he recited for me, by memory, a very fine poem by Dylan Thomas and he told me that, in 1960, he could not even have recited anything since his memory was so bad."

Expanding on the problems of the Hong Kong Veterans, Dr. Hoffer discussed a study of 100 Hong Kong Veterans vs. 50 Canadians who had served in Europe. The work was done by Dr. Richardson for the Department of Pensions in Ottawa. In contrast with the soldiers who served in Europe, the Hong Kong Veterans suffered from apathy, fatigue, insomnia, anxiety, irritability, depression, neurological and mental changes, irritable bowel, peptic ulcer, arteriosclerosis, poor dental health. The coronary death rate was about 70% higher in this group and many of them seemed to be going blind at a rapid rate, Dr. Hoffer said.

Only about 12 of the survivors, in the past 12 years, have begun the niacin therapy and they are, as far as the doctors can tell, quite normal now, Dr. Hoffer said. The 12 men have learned from each other and have thus benefited from the massive doses of the B vitamin.

"This means that we are dealing with a new category of nutritional disease which I will call an acquired dependency disease," Dr. Hoffer said. "For example, if you do not get enough niacin you get pellagra. Apparently we have about about 13 different dependency diseases. This means that a particular patient requires larger quantities of a particular vitamin than the average person so that he might require up to 1,000 times more than what is average, normal and optimal for another person.

Continued Dr. Hoffer: "It was known by the early nutritional pellagrologists that, when you were dealing with chronic pellagra, you might have to give a daily maintenance of as much as 600 milligrams of nicotinic acid per day simply to prevent those people from becoming psychotic. This was reported by our famous pioneers like Dr. Jolliffe and Dr. Sydenstricker.

"Now, when humans are deprived over a period of many years of the proper nutritional supplements, especially vitamins, that in time they are converting themselves into an acquired dependency condition. I think that what senility is, in fact, is merely a prolonged chronic form of malnutrition," Dr. Hoffer continued.

In order to stave off senility (not old age, but senility), Dr. Hoffer offered the following factors:

1. An adequate diet.

2. Adequate absorption of the nutrients in the diet.

3. Adequate circulation of the nutrients through the body.

4. Adequate utilization. There is no point getting it in if the cells cannot use it. So we have to look after our hormones and coenzymes, he said.

5. An acceleration of the process of detoxification.

"We must have enough high-quality protein; a proper balance of fats; a marked reduction in the consumption of refined sugars, especially of sucrose; and, not only should the diet be balanced over the whole day, not only should it be balanced over the meal; it should be balanced per individual food. As Dr. Roger Williams has shown by feeding individual foods to animals, you can soon recognize those foods which by themselves are totally inadequate, and which ought not to be included in any general diet. So, we have a proper dietary control," Dr. Hoffer said.

Dr. Hoffer suggested the use of supplements, particularly those nutrients which seem to be the most relevant. He listed them thusly:

"Nicotinamide, which was used in 1939 by Dr. William Kaufman, who published a book on this in 1949, where he described the results of 3 to 4 grams per day of nicotinamide on 600 cases of arthritis. The results were fantastic. He was able to reverse the arthritic changes which are so often associated with senility," Dr. Hoffer said.

"Nicotinic acid is a vitamin which is one of the wide-spectrum hypo-lipidemic agents that lowers cholesterol and lipids and is now the subject of a large-scale $55 million experiment by the United States. The results are very interesting and it seems that they will now decrease the current coronary death rate over a 4-year period about 65%. It also has, according to Dr. Edwin Boyle, Jr. of the Miami Heart Institute . . . remarkable anti-sludging properties."

"Next is ascorbic acid," Dr. Hoffer said. "I say ascorbic acid because my friend, Dr. Irwin Stone is here, and he insists it is not a vitamin. Anyway, I can assure you that it is safe. I have taken as much as 10 grams a day. We have given our patients as much as 90 grams a day and we have never seen any toxicity. I think the average dose should be 3 grams a day. I take 4."

The eminent Canadian researcher listed also pantothenic acid, vitamin E and pyridoxine as important nutrients. He stressed that there are other vital factors and that it is important to provide a proper balance of all the vitamins. He suggested that we cut down on smoking, exposure to radiation and toxic metals and that we concern ourselves with certain detoxifying mechanisms.

Dr. Hoffer drew laughter from his audience when he told them about his own supplement program. "I am taking at least 30 pills a day, including 4 grams of nicotinic acid, 4 grams of ascorbic acid, 800 units of vitamin E, 250 milligrams of thiamine, 250 milligrams of pyridoxine, vitamins A and D, calcium, and a bit of iron and a mineral supplement. I feel fine, but I may not. I do not know. I will let you know in about 40 years."

In the question-answer session, the question was asked whether or not large amounts of vitamin C can cause acidosis. Dr. Hoffer replied that he had had experience in giving as much as 80 grams of vitamin C by injection without any hint of acidosis. "I don't recommend this as routine, but that is what we have done," Dr. Hoffer said. He added that he had given patients one gram per hour, day and night, without any ill effects.

Dr. George Christakis noted that he thought that *Medical Newsletter* had mentioned that urate crystals had been found in some patients who were taking, he understood, 15 grams of ascorbic acid a day. "I think that the probability of acidosis under continued use, particularly in the elderly, where renal threshold or where renal (kidney) function might be decreased, is a possible danger."

Dr. Morris Linden, Director of the Jefferson Medical College Unit, Philadelphia State Hospital, was another speaker at the "Conference on Aging." He said that many of the patients undoubtedly came into his hospital with clinical and sub-clinical diseases of vitamin deficiency "which we partly recognized but, on the whole, failed to diagnose with specificity. I think we probably had some pellagrans among our patients."

Continued Dr. Linden: "We probably treated our patients correctly because we began to conclude from the research done on animals that, in the depleted animal and in the depleted human, pouring vitamins in by mouth is useless until the system can be replenished from within; until the chains of vitamins are reestablished. Then they can be assimilated from the gut.

"So," Dr. Linden said, "we started recommending quite a long time ago in our programs, and I think it has become a matter of commonality now in many places throughout the country, to restore vitamin content to our starved and depleted older patients. We begin with an injectible form of practically all the vitamins, including vitamin B12. We see that they get plenty of this the first several days of either institutional care or substitute for institutional care.

"Then, we put them on oral vitamins and certainly on good diets immediately," Dr. Linden said. "After a while, the parenteral (injection) route of vitamins can be greatly reduced and the patient can pretty largely rely on vitamins by mouth and a good diet—or perhaps diet alone."

When the questions were asked at the end of this session, someone asked Dr. Linden which vitamins were injected into his patients.

"All that we can get; everything that is injectible in a therapeutic form of vitamins," Dr. Linden responded. "I think some of them are a little bit painful, but we give them nonetheless into the muscles. The ones that we used at Northwestern Mental Health Clinical Center and at Philadelphia are called therapeutic vitamins. They contain vitamin A, vitamin D, vitamin E, all the B Complex that are available, plus folic acid and B12. You can get them in every city—the therapeutic vitamins for parenteral injection."

One of the penalties of getting old is hardening of the arteries in the legs and feet, which results in not enough blood getting to these parts. The feet and legs become cold. Warm socks and shoes, heating pads in bed and lined boots for outdoors become necessities as it becomes more and more impossible to keep feet warm.

An Illinois doctor, writing in the October 1965 issue of the *Journal of the American Geriatrics Society*, told of talking to one of his patients who had received a vitamin preparation for anemia. The vitamins, which were given by injection, included folic acid, plus other members of the B Complex and vitamin C. This patient had suffered for years with poor circulation in her feet and legs, but 24 hours after she got the injection, her cold feet became warmer and she had no discomfort for several days, though she was living in a moist, cold climate.

The preparation that the lady was given included 10 milligrams of thiamine, 10 milligrams of riboflavin, 75 milligrams of niacin, 5 milligrams of pyridoxine, 10 milligrams of pantothenic acid, 15 micrograms of B12 and 300 milligrams of vitamin C.

The Illinois physician decided to make a test with some other patients. He selected 15 who had complained of the same symptoms. The color of their feet was pale, the temperature between their toes was low. Some of their toes were reddish blue to dark blue. One patient had a small area of gangrene on one foot.

The patients were given the injections twice a week for three weeks. The color of the skin on legs and feet became pinker, the toes became warmer. The one patient's gangrene decreased in size. All patients said they suffered less from a feeling of coldness. In the more severe cases, the doctor found it was necessary to give the injections weekly or even two or three times weekly.

Dr. James F. Smith and Dr. James Bell of the University of Tennessee's Institute of Pathology described in the July 1971 issue of *Dental Survey* how they deal with osteitis, the painful bone inflammation that sometimes follows when a tooth is pulled. The doctor and dentist treated a group of 25 patients with their vitamin and zinc supplement. "There was a definite improvement in the majority (64%) of the patients. Another 24% demonstrated a fair degree of improved healing. No dry sockets developed in the extraction patients, all of whom had previously experienced localized osteitis," the doctors said.

The capsules that were given the patients contained 79 milligrams of zinc sulfate, thiamine, riboflavin and pyridoxine. The supplement was given on the day of the surgery and for two months afterwards.

At the Third Congress of the Italian Academy of Forensic Medicine, held in New York City in 1963, Dr. Carlo Sirtori outlined a health program that he recommends for parents-to-be. "I have always found it disconcerting that so important an event as conception should be allowed to take place without any specific prior care, considering that its effects may last, in some cases, even for centuries." Dr. Sirtori cautioned either parent from having X-rays for two months before conception. Both should be free of virus diseases for at least three months before. And he recommended liberal amounts of vitamin A, the B Complex and vitamin E. Further, he cautioned against the use of nicotine or alcohol for three months prior to conception. He added that both the sperm and the egg can be harmed by bad health habits.

In *Let's Get Well*, Adelle Davis tells how pantothenic acid is responsible for turning uric acid into harmless substances that are easily excreted by the body. If there is not enough pantothenic acid in the diet to process all the uric acid being manufactured, it will collect and cause trouble. One of these troubles is gout, the painful inflammation of the joints which usually affects the toes. A lack of vitamin E can also cause difficulty. Animals lacking in this important vitamin excrete far more uric acid than normal animals on a normal diet. And when the deficient animals are given enough vitamin E, the overproduction of uric acid stops.

Past generations have called gout a "rich man's disease" because it generally afflicted a member of the upper classes rather than a peasant or a laborer. Rich food caused it, said the medical practitioner of that age. Quite another explanation is given by Miss Davis, however. She tells us that, during those early days, the rich people ate mostly meat, since bread and vegetables were considered only good enough for the masses. Since there was no refrigeration, most of the meat was spoiled and its fat was rancid. Rancid fat destroys vitamin E almost instantaneously, so gout caused by vitamin E deficiency may have been common in those days. The poorer people who lived mostly on freshly baked black bread, rich in vitamin E and the B Complex, did not generally suffer from gout.

"For the past 30 years we have had enriched or fortified flour, breads and several cereal foods," said Dr. Elmer L. Severinghaus, Brookfield Center, Connecticut, in the February 1972 issue of *Food and Nutrition News*. This is a publication of the National Live Stock and Meat Board, Chicago, Ill. "The items added to the usual commercial foods for this purpose include only three members of the vitamin B group—thiamine, riboflavin and niacinamide, plus iron. Although such enrichment has been very important for the health of our nation, further knowledge about the vitamins has indicated a need for other members of the vitamin B group, such as pyridoxine, folic acid and vitamin B12.

"Folic acid and pyridoxine can be included in the widely used tablets or capsules of supplemental multiple vitamins," Dr. Severinghaus continued. "The daily use of such vitamins is worthwhile as nutritional insurance for those persons who do not know how to choose dietary constituents wisely, or whose circumstances of living make such choices very difficult."

"Diet and nutrition play an important role not only in caries (decay) production, but also in the rate of degeneration of the bone and gingiva (gums) supporting the teeth," said Dr. Harry Roth, a New York periodontist, in *Drug Trade News* for May 27, 1963. "Vitamin A, the B Complex, vitamin C, vitamin D, calcium, phosphorus and protein are needed for repair of alveolar bone, connective tissue and epithelium which comprise the periodontium. These nutrients are woefully lacking in many of the patients' diets."

Dr. Irwin Walter Scopp, Professor of Periodontia and Oral Medicine at the New York University College of Dentistry, said that "large therapeutic doses of the vitamin B Complex in the treatment of post-menopausal women is helpful." He added that he cannot produce proof that the unhealthy mouth conditions respond directly to the vitamins, but he knows that "the increase in vitality, cheerfulness and diminution of neurotic complaints is marked." He said further that, during and after the menopause, women customarily suffer from a deficiency in the B vitamins, which may result from just not getting enough at meals. There may also be a deficiency caused by a low level of estrogen, one of the female sex hormones.

In *Lancet* there was a discussion on how a vitamin deficiency is involved in the depression which often accompanies The Pill. Drs. Sarah A. Price and P. A. Toseland of Guy's Hospital in London say that The Pill may activate a substance which creates a deficiency in pyridoxine. These physicians say they have evidence in 20 patients that this is indeed the case. The laboratory tests showed that some women taking The Pill have in their urine certain substances that are found in the urine of people suffering from arthritis, lupus erythematosus, scleroderma, bladder and breast cancer.

"More recently," the doctors continued, "there have also been reports of symptoms and signs mimicking rheumatic arthritis and exacerbations of . . . lupus in women on oral contraceptives. On the basis of this evidence, is there not a case for routine administration of pyridoxine to all women on contractive pills or even for the inclusion of the vitamin in all . . . oral contraceptives?"

Adelle Davis, as a professional nutritional consultant, prepared special diets for patients referred to her by various doctors. Here is what she said about cataracts in *Let's Get Well.*

"My files contain dozens of unsolicited letters from persons who have recovered from cataracts after their diets were more adequate, often while they are preparing for surgery. People sometimes take only a vitamin B2 supplement and then wonder why their eyes fail to improve. An anti-stress diet high in protein, vitamin B2, vitamin E, vitamin C, pantothenic acid and all nutrients is essential before good results can be expected."

"Much of the malnutrition in this country is secondary to physical, mental or physiological stress of many kinds," said three National Dairy Council scientists in the March 1971 issue of *Geriatrics*. They went on to recount the many problems that face our senior citizens, including illness, fatigue, personal problems, loneliness, surgery, etc. Included in the discussion were some interesting observations on how the various vitamins and minerals may not be available to the older person, simply because of his diet, inability to absorb the nutrients, etc.

"Some of these long-term complications, such as vitamin B12 deficiency and metabolic bone disease, may not appear until several years after an operation," the authors said. Presumably by this time the doctors and the patient do not relate the illness to the operation, since they have forgotten the details.

At the American-Canadian-British Schizophrenia Association conference, held September 28, 1971 in London, Dr. H. L Newbold and Son-Oak Rhee, R.N., give some case histories on how vitamin B12b was used dramatically to cure mental illness. Their paper is titled, "The Use of Vitamin B12b in Psychiatric Practice." Vitamin B12b is hydroxocobalamin, a form of vitamin B12.

"Deficiencies of the B Complex vitamins—thiamine, niacin, riboflavin and vitamin B12—are associated with impaired vision," we are told on Page 93 of the USDA's "Benefits from Nutrition Research—Report No. 2." "In some instances, adverse changes in vision thought to be due to vitamin A have responded to vitamin B therapy but not to additional vitamin A.

"The B vitamin deficiencies are more likely to be associated with deterioration of vision resulting from optic nerve degeneration," the report continues. "This condition is often found in the adolescent school girl or in young adults eating a monotonous poorly balanced diet. B vitamin deficiency also is likely after periods of calorie restriction, whether deliberate or involuntary. Dimness of vision from B vitamin deficiency may be recognized with greater frequency in the future as greater demands are placed on acuteness of vision by wider education and the need for more skilled labor."

In its section on "Cosmetic," the USDA report stated: "Vitamins are the nutrients most often implicated in unhealthy appearance of the hair and skin. The skin and hair changes associated with vitamin deficiency were characterized long before the nutritional origins of the conditions were recognized. Riboflavin, niacin, pyridoxine and possibly pantothenic acid are the members of the B Complex group that have clinical dermatological significance for man," the report continued. "Vitamins A and C also are involved. Changes in skin and hair appearance with age may be partially attributable to chronic marginal intake of some of the vitamins. Pallor and skin changes are being found by Hodges and Sauberlich in ongoing studies with adults on vitamin A deficient diets."

There is hope for our senior citizens who face the possibility of loss or impairment of vision. In an article in the May 1966 issue of the *Journal of the American Geriatrics Society*, Dr. Harry Eggers, Director of Ophthalmology, St. Luke's Hospital, New York, gives a detailed discussion on the good and bad diets that may affect many old people. His excellent suggestions, of course, include the taking of vitamin supplements. He notes that arachidonic acid is the most valuable of all the unsaturated fats, but it is very scarce in food. To change linoleic and linolenic acid (both plentiful in the foods listed by the doctor) into archidonic acid, the liver must have a lot of pyridoxine. Dr. Eggers gives his patients a 50-milligram tablet of this vitamin with each meal. He also points to a need for vitamin E and these vitamins from the B Complex—inositol, choline,

B12 and niacin.

"One of the increasingly serious problems of aging is impairment or loss of central vision," Dr. Eggers said. "Such a patient may be given the dubious reassurance that he never will become completely blind but will retain peripheral (or partial) vision. This is scant comfort to a person whose chief diversions are likely to be reading, writing, painting, handicrafts or watching television. It should be emphasized that, especially in the early stages, it is possible to prevent further loss of central vision and even to obtain improvement, if treatment is started without delay."

A little over 20 years ago a laboratory experiment was performed which may have proved more about fighting fatigue than any research done since then. *The Proceedings of the Society for Experimental Biology and Medicine* for July 1951 reported on the work of Dr. B. H. Ershoff. He was feeding laboratory rats on the usual diet—the kind that sustains these animals in good health for a lifetime.

Dr. Ershoff divided his rats into three groups. The first group was given some synthetic vitamins in addition to their diet. The second group got the basic diet with all the B Complex added. The third group was fed the basic diet with 10% desiccated liver added. In other words, one-tenth of what these rats ate was highly concentrated liver. Dr. Ershoff knew that liver is a rich source of all the B vitamins, but he wanted to find out if there were possibly other things in liver that are powerful weapons against fatigue.

He then gave each group of rats a fatigue test. They were placed in a vat of water from which they couldn't escape, so they were forced to swim as long as they could. The first group of rats swam for about 13 minutes and then gave up. They were exhausted. The second group swam just a bit longer and had to be rescued.

The third group—which had been eating large amounts of concentrated liver—had almost unlimited endurance. Three of them gave up after about an hour and a half. The rest were still swimming vigorously at the end of two hours.

Dr. Ershoff had been feeding these animals liver for three months. This was no one-shot pill they had been given. Three months in the life of a rat corresponds to about 10 years in the life of a human being. So these animals had had the chance to gain full benefit from their liver supplement. And they had eaten a lot of liver every day.

Desiccated liver is liver from which all the moisture has been removed. It is entirely protein, a bit of fat and the rest is vitamins and minerals. It is doubtful that any human—except possibly a professional athlete—could manage that much liver every day. But we all need weapons against fatigue, tiredness and inertia that does not come so much from physical exertion as from nervous tension and work. Liver will help to overcome this fatigue. You should, therefore, eat liver at mealtime as often as possible, and perhaps add desiccated liver to your list of food supplements.

A physician at the Hospital for Sick Children in Toronto, Canada wrote in an article in 1968 that the "executive drinker" must begin to pay strict attention to his diet. Dr. W. Stanley Hartroft indicated that this person needs much more protein than he can possibly get in the average diet. He also needs large amounts of the B vitamins. At the time we wrote to Dr. Hartroft, asking whether or not children might be harmed by the large amount of sugar in their diets. Isn't sugar as destructive to the B vitamins, hence to the liver, as is alcohol, we inquired.

Dr. Hartroft replied that, under certain conditions, the sugar may be more harmful. "When rats are fed an amount of sugar which supplies calories equal to what other rats obtain from alcohol, under some conditions the sugar harms the liver as much as the alcohol, and, under other more carefully controlled conditions, the sugar harms the liver but the alcohol does not," Dr. Hartroft said.

On the following pages you will find lists of common foods and their content of the various B vitamins.

CHAPTER 16

Recent News About the B Vitamins

IT'S A RATHER complicated story, but it seems that a perfectly natural substance—which occurs in food along with folic acid—may have broken down some of the prejudices of cancer experts against using anything "natural" to fight cancer. A food substance is being used in the treatment of certain bone cancers. It is especially useful for children suffering from bone cancer and is being used in the treatment of Senator Edward Kennedy's 12-year-old son.

The substance is the "citrovorum factor." The way in which it helps to treat cancer is very complicated. The drug *methotrexate* has a chemical formula C20H22N8O5. It is a drug that kills cancer cells by tricking them into believing that it is folic acid, the B vitamin to which it is closely related. The cancer cells stop dividing and multiplying, which finally kills them. Cancer cells divide rapidly and wildly so any substance which can stop this proliferation can stop the progress of the cancer. But other body cells also divide and some of them divide quite rapidly, but in a controlled, healthy way. The problem is to work out some way whereby the killer drug will kill only cancer cells and will not harm normal cells.

About ten years ago, a Pennsylvania physician began to use large doses of the toxic drug to stop cancer, followed by small amounts of another drug called "citrovorum factor", which would perform as an antidote and would protect normal cells from the effects of the cancer drug. *The New York Times* for March 24, 1974, reporting on a speech at an American Cancer Society meeting, says: "Citrovorum factor, also a chemical relative of folic acid, seems to protect normal cells preferentially from the effects of methotrexate, but its precise action is not known."

At the Children's Cancer Research Foundation in Boston, doses of the toxic drug are infused into the blood of children with one kind of deadly bone cancer. Then for about three days the citrovorum factor is administered until the levels of the toxic drug are safe. This treatment is repeated every three weeks for two years.

In *Diseases of Metabolism*, edited by Garfield G. Duncan and published in 1962, the citrovorum factor is discussed at length. It consists of several elements which are closely related to folic acid. In 1948, some researchers were looking for some substance in liver which had certain effects like those of folic acid, but was not the B vitamin. They isolated the "citrovorum factor." And they showed that slices of liver could change folic acid into citrovorum factor. They reported that this factor was much more active than folic acid in producing certain results in cells.

Other researchers tested this substance in comparison with folic acid. They found that, in tropical sprue, pernicious anemia and many other kinds of blood disorders, the citrovorum factor brought relief. They gave the substance in massive amounts and encountered no adverse effects. They discovered, they say, that the amount needed by individuals might vary greatly. There is no such thing as a "standard dose."

It seems to us that the lesson to be learned here is the same lesson we health seekers preach all the time—the value of natural, whole substances as compared to fragmented, depleted, isolated, concentrated substances. The citrovorum factor is obviously something that accompanies folic acid in food. It should be taken at the same time as folic acid in a natural substance, not a synthetic substance manufactured in a laboratory. Liver and kidneys are the two best sources of folic acid and, presumably, the citrovorum factor also.

The April, 1974 issue of *Psychology Today* tells the story of a schizophrenic, 11-year-old boy and the treatment he was given which controlled the disease within several months, although his psychiatrist, Dr. Harvey M. Ross, believes the boy should continue the treatment for several years. The treatment that Dr. Ross prescribes is the orthomolecular treatment (megavitamin therapy), along with a diet to combat low blood sugar.

The child talked to phantoms he believed were in the room with him. He set fires. He attacked his sisters. He stole. Sometimes he stole candy bars. And sometimes he ate as many as 60 candy bars in one day. Says Dr. Ross, "Mitch's story, with some variations, is all too common." His parents had taken him to several psychiatrists who had not helped. One of these doctors told Mitch's parents he would not recommend megavitamin therapy "for it is too dangerous." He did not explain how it might be dangerous—more dangerous than therapy in a mental hospital, for example?

"I totally disagree with this position," says Dr. Ross in the article. "I practice orthomolecular psychiatry. This relatively young school of psychiatry believes that thoughts, emotions and actions are affected by the physical condition of the body, that the nervous system cannot be expected to perform its complicated functions unless it is provided with proper chemical milieu and that schizophrenia is the result of chemical imbalance."

After a series of tests, Dr. Ross discovered that Mitch was hypoglycemic. That is, his blood sugar regulating mechanism is disordered, so that, when he eats carbohydrates, the level of blood sugar declines, leaving his nervous system too little nourishment. Hence he suffered from the distorted perceptions (hearing, seeing, taste and smell) that torture schizophrenics.

Mitch was put on a diet very low in carbohydrate, high in protein, with small meals and frequent between-meal snacks, also high in protein. After each meal he took massive doses of some of the vitamins which have been found to be most helpful in these cases: 500 milligrams of niacin (B3), 500 milligrams of vitamin C, 100 milligrams of pyridoxine (B6), 100 milligrams of pantothenic acid, 200 International Units of vitamin E, and a multiple B vitamin tablet to furnish some of the rest of this complex. These are, of course, very large doses, especially for a child.

Within a week, Mitch's parents noticed a difference. He became calmer and more cooperattive. Dr. Ross increased the dose of niacin to 1,000 milligrams. When Mitch became nauseated, niacinamide (another form of the B vitamin) was substituted for niacin. After a month, Mitch was losing some of his overweight and his school work improved. Dr. Ross gave him an amino acid which seems to benefit brain function.

In the orthomolecular treatment of schizophrenia, daily or weekly sessions with the psychiatrist are not essential. It's the helpful chemical reactions of the body which bring about the improvement, not the psychiatrist's words. So Mitch saw Dr. Ross infrequently. Three months later his parents said the boy was doing much better. His phantoms and imaginary wrongs had disappeared. He was losing weight steadily. He could concentrate much better. Two symptoms remained—weakness when he did not eat, and bed-wetting. The first symptom is common in people with low blood sugar. The second is very common among today's children.

Dr. Ross says that about 80 percent of adult schizophrenic patients suffer from low blood sugar, which can be treated only with a diet high in protein and very low in carbohydrate, with frequent small meals so that hunger and weakness do not develop.

Skin and Allergy News for November, 1973 tells of an 8-year-old girl bothered with peculiar skin pigmentation. The mottled coloring appeared first on her fingers when she was only eight months old and gradually spread over the rest of her body. No doctors knew how or why her skin took on this coloring. No treatment brought relief. Then her doctor discovered that the child was suffering from pernicious anemia, which, as we have reported earlier, is the disease of deficiency of vitamin B12. He gave her injections of the vitamin once a month and the pigmentation disappeared within 14 months.

Specialists still do not know how the vitamin is involved in skin pigmentation, but they say that apparently this child was born with a defect in her ability to use vitamin B12. This apparently affected not just her blood, creating anemia, but also her entire body, including her skin. This story is a good example of what Dr. Roger Williams calls "biochemical individuality"—that is, the need for far greater amounts of some food element than others may need. In this case, the need was for far more vitamin B12 than the child's diet was providing.

Four Edinburgh physicians are experimenting with a form of vitamin B3 to see whether it may prove to be a beneficial aid in the treatment of certain heart attacks which might otherwise prove fatal. They report on their work in the

October 13, 1973 issue of the *Lancet.* Drs. M. J. Rowe, B. J. Kirby, M. A. Dolder and M. F. Oliver of the Royal Infirmary in Edinburgh, Scotland tell us that, in patients who have a myocardial infarction (that is a heart attack in which one part of the heart loses its blood supply), the patient always has raised levels of free fatty acids in his blood. In the case of serious disorders of the rhythm, the same thing is true.

The raised levels of fatty acids in the blood come from body fat tissue, say the authors. It is known that nicotinic acid (B3) controls this release of fats. So, these physicians theorized if they could give enough of the vitamin they might be able to control the amount of fat being released into the blood, hence improve the condition of the heart.

One form of the vitamin could not be used in large doses because of the effect it has on the heart, so they decided to use another form. First they tested the vitamin with healthy volunteers. They tested the amount of fatty acids in their blood, then gave them 200 milligrams of the B vitamin and tested their blood again every 15 minutes for the next two hours, then one hour later and two hours later. The levels of fatty substances in blood began to fall within 15 minutes after the vitamin was given. The level fell steadily for two hours, then rose again to the pretreatment level within four hours.

Then the researchers did the same test on five men who had suffered a myocardial infarct, testing their blood continuously from the time they gave them the B vitamin. The levels of fatty substances in the blood fell 50 percent from their former level. In another test of six patients with acute myocardial infarction, they gave the vitamin and tested fatty levels in the blood. "In all the patients on the drug there was a steep fall in plasma free fatty acids in the first hour, reaching a nadir during the first two hours," they say. The greatest decrease was 54 percent in one patient. In a third group of heart patients, the same thing occurred, with the greatest decrease being 58 percent. In every case the levels of fats rose again after the vitamin was discontinued.

The authors tell us they have had the same effects in animal experiments. They caution that the "drug," as they call the B vitamin, must be given every two hours to maintain the fall in fatty substances and must be given in large doses—in this case, 200 milligrams. They say they are studying the effects of the vitamin on disorders of heart rhythm.

A 53-year-old woman was brought to a Washington, D.C. hospital with lack of appetite, weight loss, lethargy, incontinence and a certain kind of anemia which causes the storage of iron in the bone marrow. The doctors consulted on her case and remembered that some kinds of anemia respond to pyridoxine (B6), given in large doses. Animals which are deficient in pantothenic acid develop anemia, but no one has apparently ever seen such anemia in a human being. However, doctors know there are nerve defects where there is a deficiency in pantothenic acid in both animals and humans.

The present victim had been ailing for months. She apparently had tuberculosis, had a poor memory, had lost 23 pounds and had fallen several times. She weighed only 81 pounds. Other doctors had diagnosed her anemia but she did not respond to iron medication.

The Washington doctors gave her large doses of pyridoxine. She did not respond. Then they tried large injections of pantothenic acid. The day after this therapy was started she was more alert, had a better appetite, a better response to stimuli and became quite cheerful. Nine days after the injections began, she was sitting on the edge of her bed, obviously greatly improved.

The doctors continued giving her increasingly large doses of pantothenic acid until she was taking 200 milligrams daily in injections. Her health continued to improve. After the vitamin injections were stopped, the improvement continued and, eventually, she was discharged from the hospital.

Five years later she was readmitted, with vaginal bleeding from an advanced cancer of the cervix, which was treated by radiation. Once again she became anemic, lethargic, had no appetite and was rapidly going downhill. Intravenous fluids were started which included 250 milligrams of pantothenic acid. She began to improve almost at once.. "After a week intravenous fiuids were no longer needed," says the article reporting on this case in *Journal of the American Geriatrics Society*, Volume XXL, No. 2, 1973. So the vitamin therapy stopped and she immediately began to grow worse. At a later hospital admission, the cancer which had been treated by radiation had invaded many other organs, she was once again anemic, mentally dull and lacking appetite. She died from cancer.

The doctor who treated her states that, despite absence of definite proof that she apparently had an anemia which responded to pantothenic acid, it seems likely that this was the case. Since she needed very large doses of the vitamin, it appears that she was not just deficient in the vitamin but "dependent" on it. This means that she needed every day very, very large amounts of this B vitamin—much larger than the average individual needs. Such a condition is "probably rare," this physician thinks, but, he says, since there are many vitamin supplements available and lots of people are taking fairly large amounts of some vitamins, perhaps the disease is much more common than physicians expect or diagnose.

The physician concludes by recommending that lethargic patients with a certain kind of anemia "might benefit from a careful trial of pantothenic acid, particularly if pyridoxine therapy has not been effective."

You will note that, throughout this entire story, not a word is said about what the poor woman had been eating all her life, which undoubtedly had a great deal to do with bringing this condition on in the first place. Let's say she was born with very large requirements for pantothenic acid or one of the other B vitamins and she was eating, every day, a diet which contained almost none of these vitamins. And she did not take vitamin supplements. How could she avoid becoming ill? And why didn't someone at the hospital teach her how to eat and what to eat and give her vitamin pills to take home? This might have prevented all her future trouble.

It is an established fact that certain disruptions of the body's use of an amino acid and a B vitamin occur during pregnancy. The amino acid is tryptophane. The B vitamin is pyridoxine. The disruption occurs during "a few months" of pregnancy according to five New York and New Jersey specialists writing in the *Lancet* for November 21, 1970.

The oral contraceptive, "The Pill," creates a false pregnancy in the body of any woman taking this drug. The false pregnancy continues for the period during which The Pill is taken. When The Pill is discontinued and menstruation induced once again, the body must readjust to not being "pregnant" any longer. But, as soon as the woman begins taking the oral contraceptive again, the same abnormal body changes begin again.

You might ask, at this point, whether doctors who have administered The Pill to many millions of women have considered the possible effects of all this disruption on the physical and emotional life of the women who take them. You might also ask why these physicians have not suggested a less harmful contraceptive, such as the "old fashioned" condom, to name one.

Therefore, it is encouraging to find that, after all these years, a few researchers are beginning to inquire into the possibility that some of the side effects of The Pill may be due to deficiency in pyridoxine, whose metabolism is so drastically changed by The Pill.

In April, 1970 the *Lancet* published a letter from two Madison, Wisconsin researchers who investigated the emotional side effects of oral contraceptives on 58 patients who had been taking the drugs for an average of 14 months. The symptoms they asked about were: irritability and emotional lability, depression, fatigue, mild paranoia (the feeling that you are being persecuted or imposed on), difficulty with sleep concentration and sleep disturbances.

Twenty-two of the patients had all five symptoms. Eight had symptoms throughout the cycle, which became worse 2-5 days before menstruation. Fifty of the patients reported that they had some of these symptoms before starting on The Pill, but the symptoms had become much worse and new emotional symptoms had appeared since starting the oral contraceptive.

The Wisconsin doctors gave their patients pills containing 50 milligrams of pyridoxine to take every day. "Of the 26 patients who showed considerable improvement, five had all five symptoms before taking vitamin B6 and only one symptom afterward. The eight patients who had no significant symptoms before taking oral contraceptives and who had at least four symptoms afterwards were all completely relieved of symptoms by pyridoxine," the authors tell us.

They go on to say, "When pyridoxine was effective the results were noticed within hours, or by the next day at the latest. The 14 patients who showed no change on 50 milligrams daily showed no improvement when the dose was increased to 100 milligrams daily. . . . Every one of the 44 patients who improved recommended pyridoxine to at least one friend or neighbor, and one friend now has 12 friends taking it. All 44 patients who improved were asked to discontinue pyridoxine to see if their symptoms returned. All refused to do so because they were so pleased with the results. Four patients who discontinued oral contraceptives because of what they read in the newspapers insisted on continuing with pyridoxine."

In the December 21, 1970 issue of *Lancet*, the New York and New Jersey researchers, mentioned earlier, report on 43 patients (33 of whom were on The Pill) who were followed through three menstrual cycles. They were given varying amounts of pyridoxine (2 to 20 milligrams daily) and tests were made to determine whether the vitamin normalized their bodies' handling of the vitamin. Up to five milligrams daily had no effect. Some of the women needed 10 milligrams daily. Others needed 20 milligrams.

The doctors tell us that, to be on the safe side, a daily tablet of 30 milligrams of pyridoxine would probably be ample for a "normal" woman. They conclude their study by saying that, since the body's use of this essential B vitamin is disrupted during "a few months" of pregnancy, the long term use of The Pill can result in a chronic and sustained derangement of this function "in a large segment of an essentially young, healthy population. In view of this ready correctability by oral pyridoxine, might it not be advisable to recommend a vitamin B6 supplement for users of The Pill?" they ask.

One answer comes in an April 28, 1973 issue of the *Lancet* in which six London scientists report on a double-blind test of women using The Pill. This is a test in which no one involved knows what is in the pill being tested. One group is given the material being tested (in this case pyridoxine); the other group gets an identical pill containing nothing of consequence. Results are carefully documented. Then the two groups are switched, and, still without anyone knowing what is in any of the pills, the women who got the vitamin get the "nothing" pill, while those who had been taking the "nothing" pill are switched to the B6. The reason for not revealing what is in the pills is so that no one will be prejudiced in his or her reactions.

These doctors tell us they have found that 80 per cent of all women taking The Pill have altered conditions in their bodies which indicate that pyridoxine is deficient (presumably due to The Pill). The other 20 per cent has been found to be absolutely deficient in the vitamin. That is, tests reveal no evidence of the vitamin anywhere in their bodies! As you remember, the minimum daily requirement for B6 for the adult female is approximately 2 milligrams.

There have been several investigations of the possible alleviation of depression in women on The Pill by taking pyridoxine, say these authors, but until now nobody has done a double-blind test. So they set up such a test, with 22 women cooperating. They gave them an official psychological test designed to reveal emotional depression. Then they gave half of the women a tablet with 20 milligrams of B6 in it which she was to take twice a day. The other group got a placebo with the same directions. The placebo is the tablet that contains nothing but a filler, so that it looks identical to the other pill. The test went on for two months. Then, without the women's knowledge, the pills were switched for the next two months.

Tests for depression were given at intervals. These include questions about anxiety, dissatisfaction, lethargy, loss of sexual desire and absolute depression. The administration of the 40 milligrams of pyridoxine over the two-month period completely corrected the body disruption of the vitamin's metabolism caused by The Pill. Tests and measurements showed this. The eleven patients who, at the beginning of the test, had no measurable pyridoxine in their bodies improved when they were given the B6. Their depression and other unpleasant emotions vanished. The women who still had enough pyridoxine in their bodies did not notice any difference.

It seems only reasonable, does it not, that these writers should recommend B6 supplements for all women on The Pill, considering that there is really no way of knowing, without a lengthy test period, how many of them are completely deficient in the vitamin. But, no. Like other scientists, these London doctors tell us that while "it is tempting to agree with these views . . . administration of large doses of pyridoxine may not be without complications."

It seems that The Pill also creates a condition where the amount of protein in the blood is lowered and pyridoxine may help out in this mechanism. Considering that many women, especially in the high population areas of the world, are on diets extremely low in protein, it is possible that this might cause even more trouble, they speculate.

It goes without saying that no one involved in any of these experiments asked any of the women what they ate. Thus, the women who were found to be entirely deficient in vitamin B6 may be in that group of individuals who have enormously high requirements for this vitamin, as is often the case.

Or, The Pill may have for them certain disruptive actions in regard to B6 which it does not have for the women who were not entirely deficient in pyridoxine. Or, it's possible that the women who were found to be entirely deficient just never eat anything which contains this essential nutrient (wheat bran, wheat germ, wholegrain products, soybeans, meat, organ meats, whole milk, corn, brewers yeast, etc.) Or they eat so little of such food that, under the stress of The Pill and the chronic state of pregnancy which it induces, the small amount of B6 in their food was simply not enough to sustain them.

There is no indication in any of the vast amount of literature we have read on The Pill that any doctor ever recommended to any woman on The Pill that she watch her diet carefully, to make sure she gets plenty of pyridoxine-rich foods or that she take a food supplement with plenty of B6 in it. We are speaking of millions, possibly hundreds of millions of women in the world who are the mothers and grandmothers of the people who will live in the future. In addition to the very disturbing evidence that is rapidly accumulating in regard to The Pill's effects on blood sugar and circulatory complications in susceptible women, we now have proof that the administration of one inexpensive, harmless vitamin would correct one body disorder brought about by The Pill, and would prevent—for perhaps half the women on The Pill—the depression, lethargy, fatigue, irritability, paranoia and insomnia which apparently trouble them.

In the February 17, 1975 issue of *The Journal of the American Medical Association*, a group of physicians reported that even in women who do not smoke, who do not have high blood pressure or migraine headaches, oral contraceptives produce more disabling strokes than in women who do not take The Pill.

The doctors caution that their figures show a relative, not absolute risk. The risk is one in 10,000. These researchers say that this must be balanced against the risk of stroke in pregnancy. And they tell us that strokes are almost unknown in pregnancy. So they are concerned that many young women are threatened with strokes, a disorder which we formerly associated almost entirely with elderly people. Yet it seems that The Pill produces a circulatory condition in otherwise healthy young women which may lead to a disabling stroke.

An article in the *Lancet* for March 8, 1975 talks about the effect of The Pill on vitamins. For some reason that no one understands, the vitamin A content of blood is raised in women who take The Pill. No one knows where such an increase comes from and whether it may pose a threat to a child conceived after The Pill is stopped. Very large amounts of vitamin A in the blood of pregnant animals have been known to cause congenital defects in their offspring. Experts do not believe this is likely to happen with human mothers, but they don't know how to explain the phenomenon of vitamin A blood increases.

Deficiency in vitamin B2 is found, says the *Lancet*, mostly in women who just don't get enough food. This would apply to women in the Third World where gross over population is making birth control mandatory and where food is very scarce among most of the people, even now. It also might apply to women in the rich and well-fed Western countries where young women are trying to exist on unwise diets to take off pounds or simply because they don't know how to choose nourishing foods. Says the *Lancet*, "There is need for more studies on the effect of oral contraceptives on riboflavin (vitamin B2) availability in large groups of women and especially those in whom overt or subclinical deficiency already exists." Amen to that.

In the case of pyridoxine (vitamin B6), there is a massive amount of evidence on the deficiency in this vitamin which is brought about by The Pill, as we have already reported. Says the *Lancet*, "Since the initial report by Rose describing alterations in tryptophane metabolism in women on oral contraceptives and biochemical evidence of vitamin B6 deficiency, more than 100 publications have confirmed the original observations and expanded them." There is a very complex relationship between several of the B vitamins and tryptophane, which is a protein.

The majority of women taking The Pill have been shown to metabolize this protein improperly, indicating that they have some deficiency in vitamin B6 and "some of these have evidence of absolute deficiency of this vitamin." The only way to overcome such gross deficiencies, says the *Lancet* article, is for the women to take 20 to 30 milligrams of vitamin B6 daily, which is about 10 times the average intake.

One researcher tested 39 women complaining of depression which was thought to be due to The Pill. Nineteen of these had absolute deficiency of vitamin B6—that is, no vitamin at all could be measured in their blood. The remainder were not so deficient. Giving 40 milligrams a day of vitamin B6 produced improvement in those women who were deficient, but no improvement in those who still had some vitamin B6 in their blood.

Impairment of blood sugar regulating mechanism by The Pill seems to us to be the single most serious side effect yet known. And this is due, as experts believe, largely to lack of vitamin B6. Giving lots of the vitamin to women who had blood sugar disorders improved the situation. Another reseacher could get improvement only when the women were very short on vitamin B6.

Perhaps most interesting of all is the fact that in one experiment women who were not taking The Pill but had disordered blood sugar regulating showed no improvement when they were given vitamin B6. But women whose disordered blood sugar was produced by The Pill did show improvement when they got much more vitamin B6.

Now, disorders of blood sugar regulation are very serious matters, as anyone knows who has diabetes, or hypoglycemia, which is the opposite of diabetes. The circulatory troubles which almost always accompany either of these two conditions are responsible for many fatalities these days. Heart attacks, strokes, blindness and a multitude of other troubles may dog the steps of the woman whose blood sugar regulating mechanism has gone awry.

Yet we find that, while some physicians are calling for supplements of vitamin B6 to be given to *all* women on The Pill, other "experts" believe that this is "not justified" at this time. It is difficult to understand such a position. The experts do not know, they say, the long-term effects of giving vitamin B6 to women. The effects of *not* giving it are obvious. We have outlined them above. Disorders of blood sugar regulation lead to health disasters. Pyridoxine in almost any amount has been shown to be completely harmless. It is water-soluble and any amount not used by the body is harmlessly excreted.

In the case of vitamin C, reduced levels of this vitamin are found in the plasma, the white blood cells, the blood platelets and the urine of women who take The Pill. The reduction may run as high as 40 percent. Even so, says the *Lancet*, these levels are above those which we encounter in scurvy. Scurvy is, of course, the disease of total vitamin C deficiency—the condition you are in just before you die of vitamin C deficiency.

So, say the experts, it appears that, to keep their levels of vitamin C "normal," women taking The Pill would have to take as much as 500 milligrams of vitamin C a day—10 times the officially recommended amount. As many of you know, many thousands of people all over the world are taking as much as 10 times this amount just to see if they can avoid colds. No harm has been reported as a result. But still the "experts" say about women on The Pill, whether or not it is advisable or necessary to take more vitamin C "cannot be answered at the present time." We suggest that such an attitude is criminal folly.

Folic acid is lacking in the blood of women on The Pill, the *Lancet* article continues. After one year on The Pill, nine percent of one group of women had pathologically low levels of this

B vitamin. After two years, 21 percent had low levels, and after four years, 42 percent had pathologically low levels. "Pathologically low levels" mean that these women are barely avoiding megaloblastic anemia, which is an often fatal disease.

Vitamin B12, whose lack produces pernicious anemia, which can also be fatal, was found to be 40 percent lower in women taking The Pill than women not taking it. None of these women as yet had the anemia which results from lack of vitamin B12. No one knows how long it may take to produce the anemia. We are not told whether these women were given vitamin B12 or were simply examined and sent home. If they were not actually put on food supplements rich in vitamin B12, this seems like negligence of the worst sort, since this vitamin is inexpensive, easy to take and perfectly safe in any amount.

In the summary of this article, written by Victor Wynn at St. Mary's Hospital Medical School in London, England, we are told once again that all women on The Pill are threatened with vitamin deficiencies created by The Pill. But, say the authors, maybe these deficiencies are just "necessary adaptations of metabolic processes and do not exemplify true deficiencies." Unbelievable!

The Pill may be a cause of migraine headaches. The Pill may impair one's defense against infections. The Pill may bring vaginal discharges, urinary tract infections, susceptibility to chicken pox and other infections, eczema, loss of sex drive, mouth ulcers, high blood pressure, gall bladder troubles, serious alterations in results of laboratory tests which may throw off diagnoses of illness. Eighteen and a half million women were taking The Pill in 1969, undoubtedly many more than that by now. Periodically some researcher gives out a press release on research on the Male Pill, but it's never any more than a press release.

And on March 5, 1975, *The New York Times* said that the development of safer methods of contraception is being seriously hampered because the multi-billion-dollar drug industry does not see any chance of making a pile of money out of a new pill before 1990 and that's too long to wait!

So go ahead and suffer, ladies. But don't take another milligram of pyridoxine or vitamin B12 or folic acid or riboflavin because nobody knows what they might do to you, says official medical authority. And it says this in spite of the fact that its own publications are bulging with evidence of the complete harmlessness of all these vitamins taken in massive doses over many years, along with massive doses of vitamin C. The drug companies just can't make any money selling vitamins, so it's up to young women to go right on suffering the evil effects of the vitamin deficiencies the profitable drugs (like The Pill) produce in a large proportion of all young American women. Such an attitude is scandalous and must be fought.

Two days before the Food and Drug Administration finally gave approval to the "morning after" contraceptive—DES—the head of the National Cancer Institute came to life miraculously and announced to the world that this pill should be banned if "necessary use of it cannot be curbed." Dr. Frank J. Rauscher, Jr., gave his testimony before a congressional committee. Earlier witnesses said the drug is already being widely used by college students and other women.

Dr. Rauscher pointed out that 220 cases have recently come to light of women who were given DES during their pregnancy. Their daughters have developed a rare vaginal cancer. It seems quite possible that many other women so treated some 20 years or so ago also passed this legacy along to their daughters. And the daughters have not yet been found to count them in this terrible toll.

And now the FDA is permitting the use of DES as a contraceptive, even though the National Cancer Institute has called for banning it. Such are the workings of bureaucracy.

The 69-year-old woman was brought to a hospital with a history of pallor, fatigue, forgetfulness and lack of energy. On the day before, she fell in her apartment and could not get up because of weakness. Hospital attendants found it difficult to awaken her. She said she ate meat daily and fresh fruit and vegetables at least three times a week. The hospital physicians gave her a complete battery of tests in an effort to diagnose her condition. There seemed to be no doubt that she was suffering from megaloblastic anemia, with diseased red blood cells and other symptoms characteristic of the anemia caused by lack of vitamin B12.

But the patient had been given an injection of vitamin B12 the week before she came to the hospital, and her blood levels of this essential vitamin were high. So something else was obviously wrong. The doctors gave her folic acid, the B vitamin closely related to B12. She began to improve at once and was soon discharged from the hospital. Tests taken six months later showed her in good health. Her mind was clear. She walked normally. Her fatigue and forgetfulness were gone.

The authors of this article, in the *Journal of the American Medical Association* for July 31, 1972 point out that there was a history of pernicious anemia in her family. They tell us of two other elderly patients whose "dementia" was cured by giving them folic acid.

The cause of multiple sclerosis (MS) is unknown. It is, according to an article in *The American Journal of Clinical Nutrition* for August, 1973, probably the most common disease of the central nervous system affecting people between the ages of 20 and 50. Symptoms of this extremely serious, debilitating disorder include: double vision, nystagmus (uncontrolled rolling of the eyeballs), stiffness and weakness of one or more arms or legs, incoordination of muscles, tremor, difficulty in speaking, convulsive seizures, paralysis of one side of the body, "pins and needles" feelings and difficulties with urination.

Beset by one or more physical and mental problems of this nature at a time when life should be at its fullest, an MS victim is understandably in desperate straits and almost completely at the mercy of the latest medical treatment which never seems to achieve much except to alleviate some symptoms for a while.

Donald A. Mitchell and Emil K. Schandl of Nova University in Florida believe they have found a possible clue to the disease which may prove to be just as helpful to the rest of us as it is to the MS patient. Their theory involves vitamin B6 and carbon monoxide. They base their theory on geographical facts and laboratory experiments. They tell us that MS is common only in Western industrialized nations and North America. It is almost unknown in South America, Eastern Europe, North Korea, China, Alaska and the Islands of the Pacific. It rarely appears among African blacks but in the U.S. it is as common among blacks as among their white neighbors.

What one environmental factor is present in all these localities where MS is common and not present in other parts of the world? Carbon monoxide pollution of the air, say the authors. It comes from automobile exhausts and from coal-burning chimneys. Carbon monoxide does its damage by attaching itself to hemoglobin, the red coloring matter of blood cells. This results in asphyxiation and death when exposure is maintained long enough. Running a car motor with the garage door closed eventually produces death from carbon monoxide poisoning. Of 21,000 cases of this kind of poisoning who were resuscitated in time, Drs. Mitchell and Schandl tell us, a number suffered a demyelinating condition. This is the same process that causes multiple sclerosis.

Animals exposed to varying amounts of carbon monoxide in the air they breathe exhibit various degrees of destruction of the central nervous system. Left in cages at various highway locations with differing degrees of traffic density, mice were found to have degenerative changes in the nervous system in proportion to the amount of their exposure to carbon monoxide.

Cigarette smoking also brings exposure to carbon monoxide which is in the smoke. More than 50 per cent of the smoke of a cigarette may be absorbed by the smoker, and of course a much smaller amount by anyone in the same room who is not smoking. Metal working industries release still more carbon monoxide into outside air. So, for some of us who must travel in heavy traffic, who smoke, who live or work close to polluting industries, exposure to carbon monoxide can be potentially very dangerous.

Now we get to the crux of the matter. It has been shown that exposure to carbon monoxide in heavily polluted air increases the body's need for vitamin B6. The researchers who performed these animal experiments warned that, "The use of vitamins in preventing pathophysiologic changes in humans suffering chronic exposure to these gases should be investigated."

Say Drs. Mitchell and Schandl, "Assume that a potential MS victim, perhaps a person with a genetically determined higher than usual vitamin B6 requirement, is exposed to carbon monoxide in his environment over a period of time and that his diet remains relatively unchanged. Under these conditions, even though he is able to maintain an apparently stable level of metabolism, there must be, by logic, a point reached at which the daily intake of pyridoxine will be insufficient to sustain this apparent metabolic need and thus a subjective symptom appears." The symptoms may be determined by what the individual's physical state and need for vitamin B6 are.

On the basis of this theory, how can we explain the fact that MS victims sometimes have lengthy remissions when symptoms are less troubling and nerve tissues seem to be repairing themselves? Perhaps the exposure to carbon monoxide has lessened, so requirements for the B vitamin are reduced. Let's say the patient stopped smoking or moved to the country, thus getting away from some of the sources of carbon monoxide which were, theoretically, greatly increasing his need for pyridoxine. Or, let's say his diet was improved to such an extent that he was now getting enough vitamin B6 to maintain good nerve function even though he was still exposed to considerable carbon monoxide. In either or both cases, enough pyridoxine might be present to allow the nerve tissues to repair themselves to some extent.

Drs. Mitchell and Schandl conclude their stimulating article by asking whether it is not possible that those of us who do not succumb to MS may be suffering other nameless, or perhaps well-defined, symptoms relating to our exposure to carbon monoxide and our lack of vitamin B6, even though our symptoms are not so disabling as those of MS victims. We have just seen, for example, how a lack of B6 affects some users of The Pill. These women and MS victims have at least two symptoms in common: mental disorders and emotional instability.

An article in the *Canadian Medical Association Journal* for June 2, 1973 tells us that vitamin B1 (thiamine) and vitamin B12 are both essential components of the myelin sheaths of nerves and spinal cord. In cases of severe vitamin B12 deficiency, destruction of these parts of the spinal cord occurs. And giving plenty of vitamin B12 corrects the condition.

Dr. H. T. R. Mount of Ottawa, Canada decided to treat MS using thiamine and liver extract, which is a rich source of vitamin B12. He began his project in 1943 and followed some of the patients for 29 years, surely a record indicating great perseverance, patience and determination. Of the 14 patients, all were below the age of 48, some had mild cases of MS, others had severe cases. Some came back for regular treatment, others did not. However, it is gratifying to note that, under the heading of "Current Clinical Status," Dr. Mount has listed five patients as clinically well, two as clinically improved, one as greatly improved, and six as improved.

Treatment consisted of thiamine injected

along with intramuscular injections of liver extract every seven to ten days for a series of 10 treatments. Then the physician evaluted the patient's progress and decided what to do next. He tells us that no patient got any worse while he was under treatment. In patients whose symptoms recurred after treatment had been stopped, he simply gave another treatment and symptoms disappeared once again. One patient had trouble with the liver injections, due to allergy. After desensitizing her, he could continue to give her the treatment. Giving the thiamine by mouth produced no results. "It would appear," says Dr. Mount, "that some persons may not absorb vitamin B1 through the gastro-intestinal tract."

Patients who had less acute cases responded better and more rapidly than those who had advanced cases. Early treatment seemed to be more important than the age of the patient. "One patient," says Dr. Mount, "now aged 55, still returns for treatment when she considers it necessary because of a lowered sense of well-being, increased fatigue, and a tingling sensation in her hands and feet. Thirty-three years after the onset of her illness and after bed confinement for two years, she is active, does her housework, walks out alone without a cane and enjoys an active social life."

Another patient, a 59-year-old man, refused

to accept the therapy until his disease had progressed to the point where he was almost totally incapacitated. He walked with great difficulty, could not write. After taking the vitamin therapy, the patient improved gradually until, at present, he uses a cane only on the street, can step up with either foot and can use a ladder. He can once again write and his manual dexterity is good.

In the case of another patient who contracted MS at the age of 43, treatment was started within six months, she recovered rapidly and had a child. Later, she became irregular in coming for treatments, and her condition worsened, but improved at once with therapy. In the case of a man who started therapy within three years after the onset of the disease, it was continued successfully without interruption and he was completely well after nine months.

A woman who was treated initially from 1962 to 1964 improved and stopped coming for treatment. By 1967 her symptoms had returned; therapy was begun again. In 1971 she again complained of fatigue, inability to work, staggering gait. She was treated again and within a few months was well and could return to work.

"My experience," says Dr. Mount, "suggests that some factor or factors in liver extract, associated with vitamin B1 can induce remyelination in patients suffering from multiple sclerosis and probably in other cases of demyelinating disease." He suggests that further tests be made in laboratories.

Many years ago another physician, Dr. E. M. Abrahamson, treated 126 MS patients with diet —the same high-protein, low-carbohydrate diet which he used with such success in treating many other conditions. He found, he says in his book *Body, Mind and Sugar*, that blood sugar levels which were too high or too low prevailed in all the MS patients. His diet corrects both conditions by regulating the levels of blood sugar.

Dr. James A. Shields believed in 1947—and probably still does—that MS resulted from lack of trace minerals in soils due to the use of commercial fertilizers rather than organic ones. Dr. Shields based his theory on the geographical distribution of MS, since it was commoner in areas where commercial fertilizers are used exclusively.

A number of scientists are working with the theory that the kind of fats eaten throughout life influence one's susceptibility to MS. Dr. Hugh Sinclair of Oxford University in England has pointed out (*British Medical Journal*, October 15, 1966) that human breast milk contains considerable quantities of certain fatty acids which are almost absent in cow's milk. He speculates that, if cow's milk is taken while the child's brain and spinal cord are growing and accumulating myelin, perhaps this may predestine some of these children to MS later in life, because the myelin would be improperly made.

Evidence from Harvard University shows inositol may function to control cholesterol and possibly prevent hardening of the arteries. The two Harvard researchers were working with gerbils, feeding them diets free from cholesterol but with added coconut oil or olive oil. The male gerbils developed high cholesterol levels. But when they were switched to safflower oil, rich in unsaturated fats, the cholesterol levels went down.

The scientists gave female gerbils similar diets. The females developed a serious intestinal condition on the first diet (coconut oil and olive oil). They lost weight, developed severe dermatitis and died after several weeks. None of these side effects was seen in the males. By adding brewers yeast or liver extract to the diet of the females, the scientists cured the female gerbils, suggesting that these two foods contain a substance which the male gerbil has plenty of in his body. Gerbils, incidentally, are rodents.

Delving further into the subject, the Harvard scientists decided that the substance is the B vitamin inositol. Adding inositol to the diet they prevented the dermatitis and the intestinal condition in the females. It is well known that the male testes manufacture inositol. So this is another indication that the missing nutrient in the females on the restricted diet was inositol, which the yeast and liver provided. Yeast and liver are the best sources of this food element.

The Harvard researchers point out that "reports such as these prove that our understanding of the pathology of nutritional deficiencies is still incomplete." It seems quite possible that what is true for the gerbils may be true for human beings as well. They also remind us that past research has shown that inositol helps to prevent hardening of the arteries.

In *The American Journal of Clinical Nutrition* for August, 1973, four physicians from the New York Medical College Metropolitan Hospital Center describe the lack of vitamin B2 (riboflavin) which they found in chronic alcoholics who were also suffering from other disorders.

It is common knowledge that chronic alcoholics usually suffer from many complications as their illness progresses. In this case, 22 alcoholics (some of whom were also heroin addicts) were studied. They ranged in age from 22 to 69 years, And they were suffering from the following conditions: disorders of the muscular tissue of the heart, seizures, acute and chronic inflammation of the pancreas, acute and chronic hepatitis, alcoholic weakening of many muscles, alcoholic liver disease, infections, bleeding in stomach and intestines, and delirium tremens. Such are the horrors of a life of alcoholism.

The doctors examined them for symptoms of riboflavin deficiency. They could find none. But they tested their blood and found that 11 of the patients were sadly deficient in vitamin B2. In general, these 11 had far more serious diseases than those who riboflavin levels appeared to be more normal. Giving the B vitamin brought blood levels up to normal within a week.

So, say the doctors, it is possible to be seriously deficient in this B vitamin without showing any of the traditional symptoms of deficiency. Some of these are as follows. The mouth is one of the first parts of the body to indicate too little B2. Cracks and fissures may show up at the corners. Lips may be sore. The tongue may have a burning sensation and may turn bright magenta. Or it may show fissures and inflammation.

Seborrhea is a symptom of B2 deficiency. This is an unpleasant skin condition involving scaly, greasy dandruff and scaly patches around the nose, ears, chest or back. The individual who lacks riboflavin cannot stand bright light. His eyes may feel scratchy or "sandy." They may burn. And if deficiency is prolonged, serious and irreparable damage may be done to the iris and cornea.

Like other B vitamins, riboflavin protects the nerves. Deficiency may produce "pins and needles" sensations, tremor, muscular weakness, vertigo. A condition called "burning feet" developed in war prisoners suffering from gross deficiency in this B vitamin. Riboflavin is essential for the stomach to produce enough digestive juices to assure good digestion.

Many years ago, when cancer research was in its infancy, a Sloan-Kettering researcher performed an experiment with laboratory rats which demonstrated the effectiveness of B2 in preventing liver cancer. He gave two groups of rats a chemical known to produce cancer. Then he gave one group of rats supplements of liver concentrate. These animals did not develop cancer, even though they were exposed to dangerous amounts of the cancer-producing chemical. The rats who had no such protection all got liver cancer.

Experimenting further, the scientist tested various food elements in liver and found that the B2 was the powerful substance which protected the rats from cancer. Then he tried large amounts of brewers yeast in their diets and got the same protection. Analyzing the yeast, he found that, once again, it was the vitamin B2 which gave the protection against the cancer-causing chemical.

A Massachusetts Institute of Technology study has demonstrated that pregnant animals which get more than average vitamin B12 have offspring which are larger, healthier and more resistant to disease than animals born to mothers who are getting only average amounts of this B vitamin. This research was reported by Dr. Paul N. Newberne and Vernon R. Young in *Nature* for March 23, 1973.

"In recent years, great concern has been expressed about the food habits of the adolescent. Information on the nutritional status and dietary intake of adolescent girls, whether pregnant or not, is limited, although studies on their food habits suggest that they have the poorest dietary habits of any age group," say two Department of Agriculture scientists in the November, 1972 issue of the *Journal of the American Dietetic Association.*

They go on to tell us that by 1962 the mothers of 19 per cent of all babies born in this country were 19 years old or younger and that all complications of pregnancy were most prevalent in this group of mothers. Studies done in 1969 showed that there are an alarming number of pregnancies in girls 15 and younger. Along with this disturbing information we now have the news that teenage girls are very likely to be deficient in both iron and folic acid.

The two researchers decided to find out what they could do about the incidence of deficiency in 114 pregnant girls from 12 to 17 who came to the University of Alabama Medical Center. Their status in regard to these two nutrients was compared to that of 40 non-pregnant girls in the same age group. The object was to see how the groups compared in relation to the supposed "requirement" of adolescents for various nutrients. The results of a three-day survey of the diets of both groups uncovered the fact that neither the pregnant nor the non-pregnant girls were getting anywhere near the amount of iron they need for good health. As for folic acid, both groups were far below the recommended levels. Since requirements for folic acid are especially high in pregnancy, the pregnant girls were in more perilous condition than the non-pregnant ones. All of them, of course, were risking a very serious kind of anemia which can be fatal, due to lack of folic acid. They were also risking iron deficiency anemia as well.

Why are many older folks anemic? The answer is given in *Geriatrics* for May, 1974, in an article by Dr. Thomas H. Jukes and Dr. Henry Borsook of the University of California. They report that anemia—several kinds of anemia—are relatively common among older folks. Not just iron deficiency anemia, but also macrocytic and megaloblastic anemia. Symptoms involve enlarged size of blood cells and deficiency of bone marrow where the blood cells are manufactured. To prevent all three kinds of anemia, say Jukes and Borsook, we must supply five nutrients: the amino acid (or form of protein) lysine, folic acid, vitamin B6, vitamin B12 and iron. And, they point out, plenty of calcium, since old people tend to have osteoporosis or bone softening, which can be prevented by plenty of calcium at mealtime. For various personal and economic reasons, our senior citizens are often badly nourished. This can lead to many disorders.

Recently, the Gerontology Research Center of the National Institutes of Child Heath and Human Development uncovered an alarming prevalence of low vitamin levels in 200 elderly men from all economic classes. One-fifth of the men who were not taking any vitamin supplements showed evidence of abnormally low levels of vitamin B1 and vitamin B2. There was also evidence of abnormality in the levels of certain enzymes which change when vitamin deficiency is present.

"To provide the recommended daily allowances of vitamins and iron (for the elderly) from food sources alone would need more calories (nearly 3,000 daily) than would be desirable. It would call for a nutritionist's knowledge of food composition, and the diet would allow so little variation that it would be monotonous, and also would be expensive. Nearly everyone can afford a good multivitamin supplement with iron," say Dr. Thomas H. Jukes and Dr. Henry Borsook.

An engrossing mystery story is told in *Nutrition Reviews* for March , 1975 by Dr. E. J. Underwood, who is one of the great authorities in minerals and trace minerals and author of *Trace Elements in Human and Animal Nutrition.* Cobalt is a trace mineral which occurs usually along with silicon, which is used to give a blue color to ceramics. Not much information there that would lead one to suspect that human beings just can't get along without cobalt—an amount of cobalt so small that it seems infinitesimal. But we must have a tiny bit of cobalt.

The need of animals for cobalt was established in the mystery story which Dr. Underwood tells entertainingly. Australian sheep and cattle began to fall prey to a mysterious illness about 50 years ago. It was called "coast disease" or "wasting disease." The animals wasted away and died, destroyed by a kind of anemia which could not be cured except by giving them huge amounts of crude iron salts and ores. Well, it's iron deficiency anemia, said the experts. But Dr. Underwood and a colleague thought it was strange that so much of the crude iron ore should be necessary to cure simple anemia. So they prepared an extract of the ores with all the iron removed. And it cured the animals' disease! So, obviously, the cure must be something else in the ore that was missing from the animals' diets —some trace mineral perhaps. And it was—cobalt.

But somebody then discovered that giving whole liver to animals also cured the wasting disease. It's the cobalt in the liver, the experts thought. They removed the cobalt from the liver and gave it to the sick animals as pure cobalt but got no results. "This led to the suggestion," says Dr. Underwood, "that the potency of liver was due to the presence of a stored factor and that cobalt functions through the production of this factor within the body" of the animals in question. In other words, the animals had to have the cobalt in order to produce something else that they stored in their livers. And it was that "something else" which cured the animals. It took 11 years for workers in labs in many parts of the world to discover that the "something else" was vitamin B12, which is the only vitamin that contains a trace mineral. That trace mineral is cobalt. You cannot make vitamin B12 without it. Human beings cannot manufacture vitamin B12, as ruminant animals can, for they have an entirely different kind of intestinal mechanism. So human beings must get their vitamin B12 in the form of a vitamin. And it must contain cobalt. According to Dr. Henry Schroeder, another specialist in mineral nutrition, only one microgram (one-millionth of a gram) of vitamin B12 "can make the difference between life and death from pernicious anemia."

It might surprise you to hear that some substances suspected of causing bladder cancer are things some of us use every day, some of us use at every meal. The June 23, 1973 issue of the *Canadian Medical Journal* contained an article on the subject by Dr. Balfour M. Mount of the Department of Urology at the Royal Victoria Hospital and the Department of Surgery at McGill University in Montreal.

There are currently some 1.8 million manmade chemicals at large in the environment and 400 new ones are introduced every year. But here are the ones now being evaluated for their possible cancer-causing qualities: pain killers that contain phenacetin, artificial sweeteners, Cyclophoshamide and chemicals which interfere with tryptophane metabolism (tryptophane is an amino acid or form of protein). Also suspected of being cancer-causing are bracken fern, tobacco, viruses and coffee.

Dr. Mount tells us that the incidence of bladder cancer in smokers is approximately twice that of non-smokers. There is the possibility that the way in which smoking causes bladder cancer is the ability of even one cigarette to lower vitamin C levels in the blood and urine. Dr. Mount adds that sufficiently high levels of vitamin C can be obtained in the urine by taking 500 milligrams of vitamin C three times a day at intervals during the day.

Dr. Mount reports that vitamin B6 tends to restore the bladder cancer victim's tryptophane metabolism to normal. About half of all patients with bladder cancer excrete elevated amounts of the breakdown products of this amino acid, which is believed to be cancer-causing.

"It seems reasonable to proceed with a prophylactic regimen of 200 milligrams of pyridoxine daily which is non-toxic and may rectify the whole metabolic picture where some cancer-causing chemicals are concerned," Dr. Mount says.

Thus we see that researchers around the world are continuing to get results with one or more of the 11 vitamins of the B Complex. It would be prudent for every reader of this book to make certain that his diet contains those foods which are good sources of the B vitamins. Brewers yeast and liver in its various forms are "musts." And, as good-sense insurance, why not supplement your diet with a B Complex vitamin and possibly individual capsules of certain B vitamins. Your health is bound to be the better for it.

CHAPTER 17

Folic Acid Prevents Anemia

SOME YEARS AGO a physician experimented on himself to find out whether the B vitamin folic acid can be manufactured in the human intestine or whether it must be obtained in food. Dr. Victor Herbert, then at Boston City Hospital, put himself on a diet from which all folic acid was removed. He did this by boiling all his food three times. The heat and moisture involved in this process virtually destroyed not only all the folic acid but most other vitamins as well.

Then he took plenty of all other vitamins in a capsule, so that any nutritional difficulties he encountered would be certain to arise from folic acid deficiency. They began very soon. After three weeks the level of folic acid in his blood was low. At the end of seven weeks the first signs of abnormality in his blood appeared. After he had been on the deficient diet for 16 weeks, he became sleepless, forgetful and increasingly irritable. He lost weight. By the 19th week his bone marrow showed unmistakable changes in the cells, indicating absence of folic acid.

He took some folic acid in a tablet. Within 48 hours his bone marrow tests returned to normal, his mental symptoms cleared up. He believes that this test proves that human beings must get folic acid in their meals or they will eventually develop the perhaps fatal anemia that characterizes this deficiency. Not many of us boil our food three times in an effort to induce a deficiency of folic acid. But, as you think over the diets of your friends and neighbors, perhaps you have observed some which qualify as diets very low in folic acid. The vitamin is easily destroyed by both boiling and sunlight.

Other symptoms of the anemia which occurs when folic acid is lacking are these: weakness, loss of appetite, diminished vigor. Also digestive disturbance—flatulence, impaired absorption of food, and diarrhea. Skin and tissues of the mouth, gums, tongue and eyes are pale. Eventually there is breathlessness, fatigue and, because of the reduced number of oxygen-carrying red blood cells, heart damage and eventual death.

A little dose of folic acid can end all these symptoms very quickly.

Alcoholics suffer from deficiency in folic acid. In some startling experiments, Dr. Herbert and a colleague tested alcoholic patients by giving them a few drinks in the hospital. First they cured the anemia of the alcoholics, then they gave them daily doses of alcoholic drinks. Within 10 days the bone marrow symptoms of folic acid deficiency appeared again. The physicians gave folic acid. It did no good, so long as the men went on drinking. By discontinuing the alcohol or by giving *very large* doses of folic acid the physicians could prevent the anemia from returning. They finally got to the point where they could tell exactly how much alcohol every day would result in severe impairment of bone marrow. They believe that one reason alcoholics improve in a hospital is that alcohol is unavailable and folic acid *is* available in the hospital diet.

Arthritis patients have been found to be lacking in folic acid. Diets that are not nourishing, increased need for folic acid because of the arthritis or possibly increased demand because of the aspirin taken by the patient may be reasons for this. No one knows. Patients with many kinds of skin disorders are also found to be deficient in folic acid.

But pregnant women are most likely to show

this deficiency. Apparently the unborn child uses up whatever folic acid is available in the mother and the health of the mother suffers. We are told that studies of folic acid lack in pregnancy may explain many cases of "spontaneous" abortions, miscarriages and hemorrhaging in pregnancy. No one is certain whether the deficiency in folic acid is only one part of a disturbed state of health or whether it is the folic acid deficiency that directly triggers the health disasters.

One London physician stated that about 60 percent of all pregnant women are unable to meet the demands for folic acid in pregnancy. He based his conclusions on studies of 154 pregnant women. Those who were also deficient in iron suffered the most. The iron deficiency sometimes concealed the lack of folic acid. Sometimes giving folic acid prevented both deficiencies. The pregnant women's anemias responded quickly to injections of folic acid given every other day for six doses.

By 1969 the *Journal of the American Medical Association* was printing articles on folic acid deficiency in women on The Pill. By 1973 the *Journal* reported megaloblastic changes in women on The Pill in the lining of the cervix, similar to those found in folic acid deficiency. Nineteen per cent of 115 women taking The Pill had these symptoms—of "severe" folic acid deficiency. Such changes were not observed in other women on The Pill. Examining the blood of these women did not disclose any apparent deficiency. It seemed to be localized in the tissues of the cervical area.

The authors of the *Journal* article point out that changes such as they found in the cervix of their patients are sometimes mistaken by doctors for pre-cancerous changes. But just giving folic acid repaired the damage in a short time. Seventeen to 21 percent of their patients had low levels of folic acid in their blood, but, they say, women who do not have these typical stigmata also have low levels of folic acid in their blood.

They say that there are strong associations between folic acid and sex hormones. It's possible, they say, that oral contraceptives act to cause the body to use up its store of folic acid more rapidly and this is why so many women taking The Pill are short on this important B vitamin. Women who get serious anemia from the folic acid lack following The Pill may be extreme instances of a body condition which is apparently much more prevalent when it is localized in the cervix.

The Lancet for April 14, 1973 tells us that infants have far greater need for folic acid than adults. Premature babies are thought to need about 10 times more folic acid than adults. So early childhood is a time when folic acid deficiencies are very likely to show up, says the *Lancet* editorial. Premature babies tend to develop megaloblastic anemia when they are from 6 to 8 weeks old. Perhaps they should be getting this B vitamin routinely, say the authors.

Other children are also at risk from this kind of deficiency. Babies who develop digestive problems, pneumonia or some other infection, those who have iron deficiency anemia, or scurvy or conditions of malnutrition are more apt to suffer, too, from folic acid lack. They point out that an exclusive diet of goat's milk may produce such a condition since goat's milk has less folic acid than cow's milk. Children on special diets, those with diseases that reduce their appetites or their absorption of food, or diseases which increase their need for folic acid—all these may show evidence of deficiency.

Here are some conditions that produce such deficiency: sickle-cell anemia, *thalassemia major*, hereditary *spherocytosis*, and celiac disease. Testing for folic acid deficiency is a good test for celiac disease. Epileptics taking anti-convulsant drugs are also at high risk when it comes to folic acid. Heart disease in children may produce folic acid deficiency. Congenital or rheumatic heart disease are two of such conditions in which deficiency is often found. Apparently low levels of folic acid may harm the brain, so it is wise to discover the deficiency early and give the vitamin, say the authors.

The amount of folic acid you can get in a food supplement is limited by the FDA because of a peculiar quirk in its relationship to vitamin B12. Lack of either of these vitamins produces a similar kind of anemia. The anemia caused by lack of vitamin B12 produces some serious nerve symptoms which are not caused by lack of folic acid. So if the doctor apparently cures the anemia by giving folic acid, a deficiency in vitamin B12 may still continue and destroy nerve tissues before it is discovered. It seems obvious that the best way to prevent this is to supply supplements which contain both vitamins. But the easy, practical way is never the way doctors and the FDA decide to do things.

CHAPTER 18

Some Incidental Notes On B Vitamins

A PROTECTIVE CHARACTERISTIC of riboflavin (vitamin B2) was discovered and reported in the *Journal of Nutritional Science and Vitaminology,* volume 20, No. 4, 1974. Laboratory experiments revealed that it protects the liver against potential harm from carbon tetrachloride, a solvent which is used in cigarette lighters, cleaning fluid and so on. It would seem wise for people exposed to this poison at work or at home to be sure they are getting enough riboflavin.

Pyridoxine (vitamin B6) was given to a group of pregnant women to see what the results would be on the condition of their teeth. One group of women took 20 milligrams of the vitamin daily, while another group had no vitamin supplementation. Their drinking water was not fluoridated. The women who took the B vitamin had a smaller increase in decayed and missing teeth than those who took no vitamin.

A London physician uses vitamin B12 to treat psoriasis. Dr. E. Lipman Cohen remarked on another physician's letter to the *British Medical Journal*, in which the former doctor said he had tried shots of B12 for psoriasis and they didn't work. Dr. Cohen said he gives his patients a total of 30 injections. He has never found a smaller number to be of any use. "Improvement is often delayed until up to six weeks after stopping treatment," he says. No doctor should give up on this therapy until they have used his dosage (1,000 micrograms) for 30 injections.

Nutrition, Vol. 28, No. 3, 1974 carried an article on mental illness and nutrition. It reviewed four conditions in detail: epilepsy, depression, schizophrenia and alcoholism. It concluded that nutritional disorders in epilepsy may be iatrogenic—that is, caused by the treatment doctors give which destroys folic acid and vitamin D. Or epilepsy nutritional disorders may be due to abnormally high requirements for vitamin B6. In depression, said the author, Dr. J. W. T. Dickerson, the dietary deficiency may also be induced by a pill—in this case, the oral contraceptive pill which destroys vitamin B6. Or the depression may result from a dietary deficiency of potassium or thiamine (vitamin B1).

The victim of schizophrenia may be suffering from an inherited defect in metabolism and plain malnutrition may be secondary to this. In alcoholism, says this author, secondary malnutrition is the prominent factor. That is, the alcohol gradually takes the place of food. The more alcohol one drinks the more deficient he becomes in many nutrients, chiefly those of the B Complex of vitamins.

A 1974 report in *Internal Medicine News* for February 15 relates the incidence of organic brain disorders and nerve disorders in a group of patients who were found to be deficient in folic acid. These symptoms were in addition to the anemia or the alcoholism which were also present. The Yale researchers came to the conclusion that just plain folic acid deficiency can cause nerve and brain damage. A higher incidence of nerve disorders of all types was found in those alcoholics who were deficient in this B vitamin.

There appears to be a relationship between cyanide poisoning and the amount of vitamin B12 available to counteract it. According to a letter to the editor of the *Lancet* for September 15, 1973, exposure to cyanide reduces the vitamin B12 content of the liver, which is the body's detoxifying organ. Smokers and vegetarians have lower blood levels of vitamin B12 than non-smokers and non-vegetarians. Tobacco smoke contains 1,500 parts per million of cyanide. This suggests that smokers may need far more vitamin B12 than the rest of us to counteract the ill effects of the cyanide in the smoke. It has been recommended for many years that vegetarians assure themselves of a source of ample vitamin B12, since this is almost completely absent from all foods of vegetable origin. Taking vitamin B12 tablets would seem best for total vegetarians, since these are made from yeast fermentations and contain no animal products at all.

The International Journal of Vitamin Research, Vol. 39, No. 1, 1969, reported that the blood of pregnant women contains far less biotin than that of non-pregnant women. And there is a progressive fall in biotin as pregnancy progresses. Says the author, a need for evaluation of biotin as a constituent of vitamin supplements in pregnancy and other stressful conditions is indicated.

Bibliography

Abrahamson, E. M. and A. W. Pezet, *Body, Mind and Sugar*, Holt, Rinehart and Winston, New York, 1951.

Adams, Ruth, *The Complete Home Guide to All the Vitamins*, Larchmont Books, New York, 1972.

Adams, Ruth and Frank Murray, *Megavitamin Therapy*, Larchmont Books, New York, 1973.

Adams, Ruth and Frank Murray, *The Good Seeds, the Rich Grains, the Hardy Nuts for a Healthier, Happier Life*, Larchmont Books, New York, 1973.

Adams, Ruth and Frank Murray, *Vitamin C, the Powerhouse Vitamin*, Larchmont Books, New York City, 1972.

Adams; Ruth and Frank Murray, *Vitamin E, Wonder Worker of the 70's*, Larchmont Books, New York City, 1971.

Bicknell, Franklin and Frederick Prescott, *Vitamins in Medicine*, Lee Foundation for Nutritional Research, Milwaukee, Wisconsin, 1942.

Cheraskin, E. and W. M. Ringsdorf, Jr., *New Hope for Incurable Diseases*, Exposition Press, Jericho, New York, 1971.

Davis, Adelle, *Let's Get Well*, Harcourt, Brace and World, New York, 1965.

Ellis, John M., *Vitamin B6, the Doctor's Report*, Harper and Row, New York, 1973.

Heinz Handbook of Nutrition, McGraw-Hill Book Company, New York, 1959.

Hoffer, Abram and Humphrey Osmond, *How to Live with Schizophrenia*, University Books, Secaucus, N.J., 1974.

Recommended Dietary Allowances, Seventh Edition, 1968, Publication 1694, National Academy of Sciences, Washington, D.C.

Rosenberg, Harold, *The Doctor's Book of Vitamin Therapy*, G. P. Putnam's Sons, New York, 1974.

Williams, Roger J., *Nutrition Against Disease*, Pitman Publishing Corporation, New York, 1971.

Thiamine (Vitamin B1) Content of Some Common Foods

Food	*Milligrams*
Almonds, 1 cup	0.34
Asparagus, 1 cup	0.23
Avocados, 1 cup	0.16
Beans, Lima, 1 cup	0.22
Beef heart, 3 oz.	0.23
Beef and vegetable stew, 1 cup	0.12
Brazil nuts, 1 cup	1.21
Bread:	
Cracked wheat, 1 lb.	0.53
Cracked wheat, 1 slice	0.03
French, enriched, 1 lb.	1.26
Italian, enriched, 1 lb.	1.31
Rye, 1 lb.	0.81
Rye, 1 slice	0.04
Pumpernickel, 1 lb.	1.05
White, enriched, 1 lb.	1.13
White, enriched, 1 slice	0.06
Whole wheat, 1 lb.	1.17
Whole wheat, 1 slice	0.06
Cashew nuts, 1 cup	0.49
Collards, 1 cup	0.15
Cowpeas (or Black-eyed peas), 1 cup	0.41
Dandelion greens, 1 cup	0.23
Dates, 1 cup	0.16
Flour, whole wheat, 1 cup	0.66
Grapefruit juice, frozen, 1 can	0.29
Grapefruit juice, dehydrated, 1 can	0.41
Grape juice, 1 cup	0.11
Ham, smoked, 3 oz.	0.46
Ham, boiled, 2 oz.	0.57
Liver, beef, 2 oz.	0.15

Food	*Milligrams*
Milk, dry, whole, 1 cup	0.30
Milk, dry, nonfat, 1 cup	0.28
Oatmeal, 1 cup	0.22
Orange, 1	0.11
Orange juice, frozen, 1 can	0.63
Orange and grapefruit juice, frozen, 1 can	0.47
Oysters, raw, 1 cup	0.30
Peanuts, roasted, 1 cup	0.47
Peas, green, 1 cup	0.40
Pecans, 1 cup	0.93
Pineapple, raw, 1 cup	0.12
Pineapple, canned, crushed, 1 cup	0.20
Pineapple juice, 1 cup	0.13
Pork chops, 2 to 4 oz.	0.60
Pork roast, 1 slice	0.71
Raisins, 1 cup	0.13
Sausage, Bologna, 8 oz.	0.36
Soup, bean, 1 cup	0.10
Soybeans, 1 serving	1.07
Soybean flour, 100 grams	0.82
Spinach, 1 cup	0.14
Tangerine juice, 1 cup	0.14
Tangerine juice, frozen, 6 oz. can	0.43
Walnuts, black or native, 1 cup	0.28
Walnuts, English, 1 cup	0.33
Watermelon, 1 wedge	0.20
Wheat germ, 1 cup	1.39
Yeast, brewer's, 100 grams	9.69

Riboflavin (Vitamin B2) Content of Some Common Foods

Food	*Milligrams*
Almonds, 1 cup	1.31
Apricots, 1 cup	0.24
Asparagus, 1 cup	0.30
Avocados, 1 cup	0.30
Beef, hamburger pattie, 3 oz.	0.18
Beef, heart, 3 oz.	1.05
Beef, steak, 3 oz.	0.16
Beef, corned, 3 oz.	0.20
Bread:	
Cracked wheat, 1 lb.	0.42
Cracked wheat, 1 slice	0.02
French, enriched, 1 lb.	0.98
Italian, enriched, 1 lb.	0.93
Rye, 1 lb.	0.33
Rye, 1 slice	0.02
Pumpernickel, 1 lb.	0.63
White, enriched, 1 lb.	0.77
White, enriched, 1 slice	0.04
Whole wheat, 1 lb.	1.03
Whole wheat, 1 slice	0.05
Broccoli, 1 cup	0.22
Buttermilk, 1 cup	0.44
Cashew nuts, 1 cup	0.46
Chicken, broiled, 3 oz.	0.15
Chile con carne, w/o beans, 1 cup	0.31
Collards, 1 cup	0.46
Dandelion greens, 1 cup	0.22
Dates, 1 cup	0.17
Egg, raw, 1	0.15
Egg, scrambled (w/milk and fat)	0.18
Flour, whole wheat, 1 cup	0.14

Food	*Milligrams*
Kale, 1 cup	0.25
Lamb chop, 4.8 oz.	0.24
Liver, beef, 2 oz.	2.25
Mackerel, 3 oz.	0.23
Milk, whole, 1 cup	0.42
Milk, nonfat, 1 cup	0.44
Milk, dry, whole, 1 cup	1.50
Milk, dry, nonfat, 1 cup	1.44
Mushrooms, 1 cup	0.60
Mustard greens, 1 cup	0.25
Oysters, 1 cup	0.39
Peaches, 1 cup	0.32
Peas, green, 1 cup	0.22
Prunes, cooked, 1 cup	0.18
Pumpkin, 1 cup	0.14
Sausage, Bologna, 8 oz.	0.49
Shad, baked, 3 oz.	0.22
Soybeans, 1 serving	0.31
Soybean flour, 100 grams	0.34
Spinach, 1 cup	0.36
Squash, winter, baked, 1 cup	0.31
Strawberries, raw, 1 cup	0.10
Turnip greens, 1 cup	0.59
Watermelon, 1 wedge	0.22
Wheat germ, 1 cup	0.54
Yeast, brewer's, 100 grams	5.45
Yogurt, 1 cup	0.43

Niacin (Vitamin B3) Content of Some Common Foods

Food	*Milligrams*
Almonds, 1 cup	5.0
Apricots, dried, 1 cup	4.9
Avocados, 1 cup	2.4
Beef, 3 oz. portion	3.1
Beef, hamburger pattie, 3 oz.	4.6
Beef, steak, 3 oz.	4.0
Beef, corned, 3 oz.	2.9
Beef, heart, 3 oz.	6.8
Beef and vegetable stew, 1 cup	3.4
Bread:	
Cracked wheat, 1 lb.	5.8
Cracked wheat, 1 slice	0.3
French, enriched, 1 lb.	11.3
Italian, enriched, 1 lb.	11.7
Rye, 1 lb.	6.4
Rye, 1 slice	0.3
Pumpernickel, 1 lb.	5.4
White, enriched, 1 lb.	10.4
White, enriched, 1 slice	0.5
Whole wheat, 1 lb.	12.9
Whole wheat, 1 slice	0.7
Chicken, broiled, 3 oz.	10.5
Collards, 1 cup	3.2
Crabmeat, 3 oz.	2.1
Dates, 1 cup	3.9
Flour, whole wheat, 1 cup	5.2
Ham, smoked, 3 oz.	3.5
Lamb chop, 1	5.4

Food	*Milligrams*
Liver, beef, 2 oz.	8.4
Mackerel, 3 oz.	6.5
Mushrooms, 1 cup	4.8
Oysters, 1 cup	6.6
Peanuts, roasted, 1 cup	24.6
Peaches, dried, 1 cup	8.4
Peas, green, 1 cup	3.7
Pork chop, 1	3.6
Salmon, 3 oz.	6.8
Sausage, Bologna, 8 oz.	6.0
Shad, 3 oz.	7.3
Soybeans, 1 serving	2.3
Soybean flour, 100 grams	2.6
Swordfish, 3 oz.	9.3
Tuna, 3 oz.	10.9
Veal cutlet, 3 oz.	4.6
Wheat germ, 1 cup	3.1
Yeast, brewer's, 100 grams	36.2

Pyridoxine Content of Some Common Foods

(We list micrograms per serving of 100 grams, which is a bit more than 3 ounces. Remember that foods like blackstrap molasses and brewer's yeast are used in much smaller amounts than this. Even so, their pyridoxine content is remarkable).

	Micrograms
Bananas	320
Barley	320-560
Beef	230-320
Cabbage	120-290
Cod	340
Corn, yellow	360-570
Cottonseed meal	1,310
Eggs	22-48
Flounder	100
Ham	330-580
Heart, beef	200-290
Kidney, beef	350-990
Lamb	250-370
Liver, beef	600-710
Malt extract	540
Milk, whole	54-110
Milk, dry	330-820
Milk, dry, skim	550
Molasses, blackstrap	2,000-2,490
Peanuts	300
Peas, fresh	50-190
Peas, dry	160-330
Pork	330-680
Potatoes	160-250
Rice, white	340-450
Rice, brown	1,030
Salmon, canned	450
Salmon, fresh	590
Sardines, canned	280
Soybeans	710-1,200

	Micrograms
Tomatoes, canned	710
Tuna, canned	440
Veal	280-410
Wheat bran	1,380-1,570
Wheat germ	850-1,600
White flour	380-600
Yams	320
Yeast, brewer's	4,000-5,700

Vitamin B12 Content of Some Common Foods

(We give the number of micrograms in 100 grams, the average serving)

	Micrograms
Beef, kidney	18-55
Beef, liver	31-120
Beef, round	3.4-4.5
Bread, whole wheat	0.2-0.4
Cheese, American	0.6
Cheese, Swiss	0.9
Egg, 1 whole	0.3
Fish, haddock	0.6
Fish, sole	1.3
Ham	0.9-1.6
Milk, whole	0.3-0.5
Milk, powdered	1-2.6
Soybean meal	0.2

Pantothenic Acid Content of Some Common Foods

(We give the milligram content of one serving, about 100 grams)

Food	*Milligrams*
Brains (all kinds)	2.6
Broccoli	1.17
Bulgur	0.660
Cabbage juice	1.1
Cashews	1.3
Cauliflower	1
Chicken	1
Chickenpeas	1.25
Cottonseed flour	4.320
Eggs, whole	1.6
Filberts	1.146
Flounder	0.850
Heart	3
Turkey	2.67
Kale	1
Kidneys	4
Lentils	1.3
Liver	8
Mushrooms	2.2
Oatmeal	1.5
Peanuts	2.8
Peas, dry	2
Rice, Brown	1.1
Salmon	1.3
Liverwurst	2.7
Sesame seed flour	2.7
Soybeans	1.7
Sunflower seeds	1.4
Walnuts	0.900
Wheat bran	2.9

Food	*Milligrams*
Wheat germ	1.2
Whey, dried	4
Yeast, brewer's	12

Biotin Content of Some Common Foods

(We give the microgram content of a serving, which is a bit more than 3 ounces).

	Micrograms
Bananas	4
Beans, dried limas	10
Beef	4
Cauliflower	17
Corn	6
Eggs, whole (2)	25
Filberts	16
Halibut	8
Hazel nuts	14
Liver, beef	100
Milk (1 cup)	5
Mushrooms	16
Oysters	9
Peanuts	39
Pork	7
Salmon	5
Strawberries	4
Wheat, whole	5
Yeast, brewer's (3 tablespoons)	75

Folic Acid Content of Some Common Foods

(We list micrograms per serving of 100 grams)

	Micrograms
Almonds	46
Apricots, fresh	3.6
Apricots, dried	4.7
Asparagus	89-140
Avocadoes	4-57
Barley	50
Beans, Lima, fresh	10-56
Beans, Lima, dry	100
Beans, Navy, dry	130
Beef, round steak	7-17
Beef, liver	290
Beef, kidney	58
Blackberries	6-18
Bread, rye	20
Bread, wheat	27
Bread, white	15
Broccoli	34
Brussels sprouts	27
Buttermilk	11
Cabbage	6-42
Cauliflower	29
Cheese, cheddar	15
Cheese, cottage	21-46
Coconut	28
Corn, sweet	9-70
Dates	25
Egg, 1 whole	5.1
Egg, yolk	13
Endive	27-63
Flour, enriched white	8.1
Flour, rye	18
Flour, whole wheat	38

	Micrograms
Ham, smoked	7.8
Kale	50.9
Lentils, dry	99
Lettuce	4-54
Liver, beef	290
Liver, chicken	380
Liver, lamb	280
Liver, pork	220
Mushrooms	14-29
Oats	23-66
Peanuts	57
Peas	5-35
Potatoes	2-130
Rice, brown	22
Spinach	49-110
Tangerines	7.4
Turnip greens	83
Watercress	48
Wheat	27-51
Zucchini	11

Index